HOW TO NEVER LOOK FAT AGAIN

Over 1,000 Ways to Dress Thinner— WITHOUT DIETING!

New York Times Bestselling Author of *How Not to Look Old*

CHARLA KRUPP

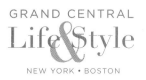

GRAND CENTRAL
Life & Style
NEW YORK • BOSTON

DEDICATED TO:

My husband, Richard Zoglin, who never gains a pound.

Grand Central Life & Style
Hachette Book Group

237 Park Avenue, New York, NY 10017
www.HachetteBookGroup.com

Printed in China
Originally published in hardcover by Hachette Book Group.
First Trade Edition: March 2011
10 9 8 7 6 5 4 3 2 1

Grand Central Life & Style is an imprint of Grand Central Publishing.
The Grand Central Life & Style name and logo are trademarks of Hachette Book Group, Inc.

The Library of Congress has cataloged the hardcover edition as follows:
Krupp, Charla.
How to Never Look Fat Again: over 1,000 ways to dress thinner—without dieting
/ Charla Krupp.—1st ed.
p. cm.
ISBN 978-0-446-54747-5
1. Clothing and dress. 2. Overweight women—Clothing. 3. Beauty, Personal. 4. Fashion. I. Title.

TT507.K78 2010
746.9'2—dc22   2009024235

ISBN 978-0-446-54746-8 (pbk.)

Design by Hoffman Creative

→ So how are those high-fat and no-fat looks going? After my tour of twenty-one cities showing women all over this country how easy it is to look THINNER BY DINNER(!), I settled in for a few months testing well over 400 beauty and body products, shapewear, bras, and workout gear along with my beauty-savvy magazine editor friend, Brette Polin. I needed to see if the newer versions of all the original brilliant buys in the hardcover edition of *How to Never Look Fat Again* were in fact better than all the products that have launched since that book hit the printer. As a result of all that dabbing and schmearing and inspecting my face and body for results, I'm introducing you to over 125 new products in this updated edition of *How to Never Look Fat Again.* I'm thrilled to tell you that in the new version you're holding, there are over 100 products under $25!

Why? Because in this economy, finding a beauty product that performs miracles for over $100 isn't as exciting as finding one that will do the same for less. I don't care how much money you have, every woman I know wants to pay less and get more. So, in judging these brilliant buys, price mattered. If two products were equally as effective, the less expensive one was the winner. But, of course, the ultimate winner in all this is you! If you already own the hardcover, you are going to save money by picking up this paperback, too!

The new message in this updated edition of *How to Never Look Fat Again* is: *Don't be loyal to products.* Loyalty to people is a virtue; loyalty to beauty products and fashion items can make you look old—and

fat! Your personal style is constantly evolving, and your products need to evolve, too. Say your favorite lipstick is discontinued. Are you one of those women who chase down whatever remaining tubes are left on the planet? If so, better to save your precious energy and just embrace the change as a signal from the universe to move on to another shade. In the world of beauty, newness most of the time benefits you as it's usually an upgrade in efficacy, ingredients, formulations, or delivery system. Unless, of course, it's the same old product with an upgraded price tag!

I still believe that a change of makeup and skincare products can make a difference. I've seen it firsthand. My sister, Lora, who lives a very casual lifestyle in California, came to New York City to visit me and we spent a lot of time testing new beauty products. When she got on the plane to go home, she looked so radiant, as if she had done something much more dramatic than try out new exfoliators, moisturizers, serums, foundations, blush, eyeliner, brow filler, mascara, and lipstick. When she got home, her friends demanded that she tell them what she did at my New York derm, to get her skin so glowing. No one could really believe that it was simply a change of products! So have fun checking out these new brilliant buys with your sister, friends, book club group . . . It's all about sharing the wealth with women you love. Let me know what new products you are obsessed with at charlakrupp.com. Here's to everyone looking younger, sexier, thinner, better by tonight!
XX,
Charla

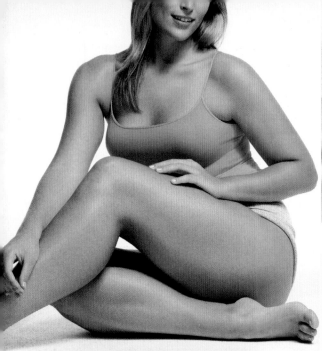
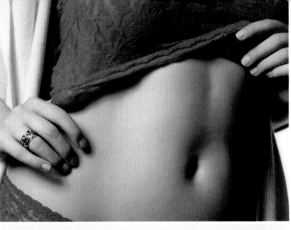
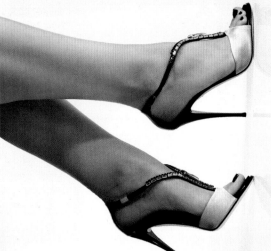
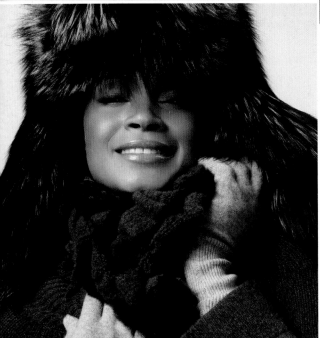
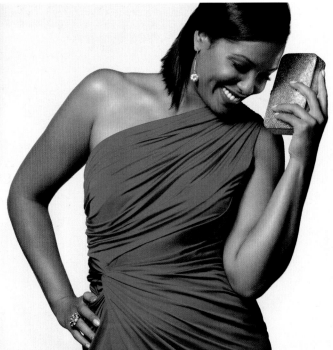
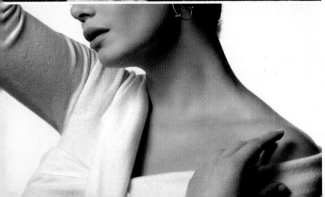

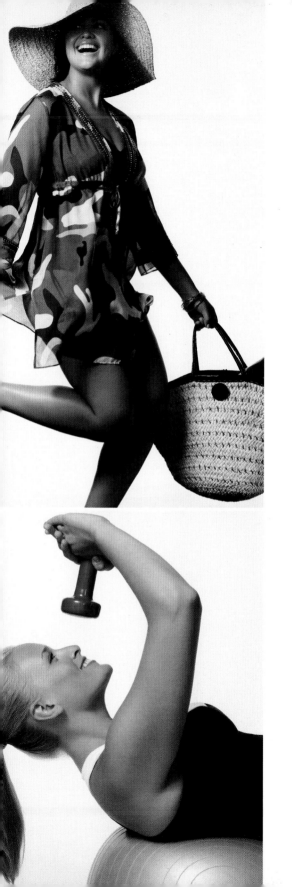

Contents

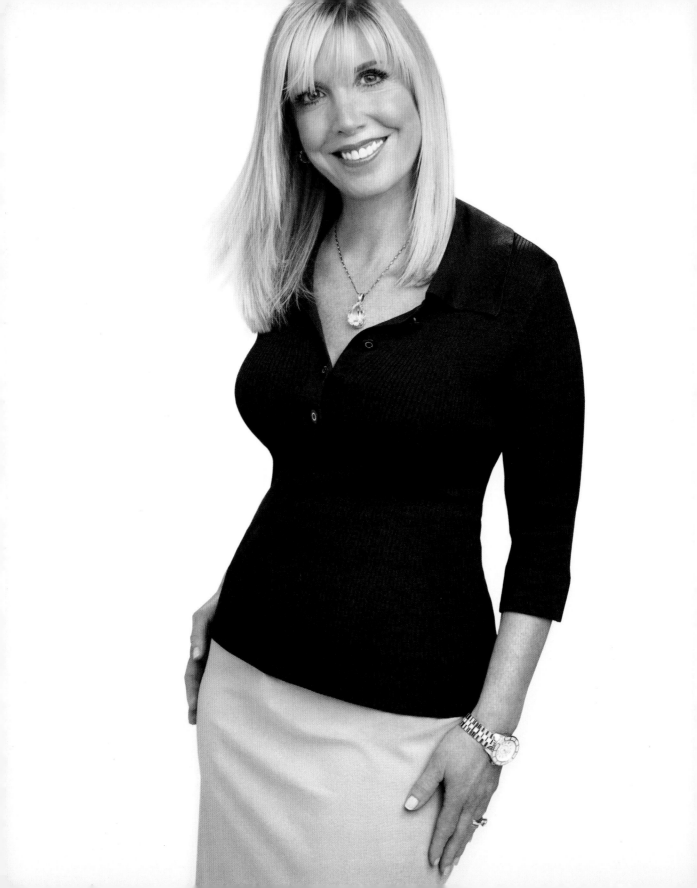

Raise Your Hand If You Think You Look Fat

YOU'RE NOT ALONE.
Almost every woman I know thinks she looks fat—even women who exercise every day, eat nothing but salads and salmon, and wear a size 6 or less!

The truth is, I think I'm fat, too. I can't stand that I've gained weight. In this past year, I have weighed many more pounds than I'd like to. As women, I think that we all carry three different weight numbers around in our head: the number of pounds we would love to weigh (in our dreams), the number we can live with comfortably, and then the number that makes us feel like we are fat. I'm sure you know what I mean. I know my numbers; you know yours. And even though the number that makes me feel fat is still within the normal healthy range for a person of my height (five feet), those extra pounds make a huge difference in how I feel, how I approach the world, and I how I dress that day.

→ What's worse—it's getting harder and harder for me to keep my weight down than it was a few years ago. I'm trying—really, I am—because this creeping poundage cannot continue with every passing year. At least that's what I tell myself.

The good news is that even though *I* think I'm fat, most other people don't. They don't see the way my middle now divides into three sections. They would never know that my favorite jeans hardly zip up anymore—or that when I do try to zip them, a bulge squeezes out over the waistband. They don't know that I've had to increase my cup size; or that my upper arms, when not under wraps, jiggle; or that cellulite lurks beneath that high-waist, long-legged piece of shapewear.

If you don't see all that, it's because I've become an expert at hiding the fat. Not by dieting and exercise—though I'm a fervent believer in both—but by wearing the right clothes in flattering fabrics, colors, and shapes and styling them with distracting accessories; by having the best supportive bra that lifts me up and gives me a couple extra inches of torso; by wearing the highest heels I can comfortably stand in; and by holding my head high, my shoulders back, and being aware of my posture. I've gathered more than a thousand tips like these that go way beyond curating a closetful of black—which is not only depressing but fools no one.

I knew some of this from thirty-plus years of editing fashion magazines (*Glamour, InStyle, People: StyleWatch, Shop Etc.*), directing the beauty coverage for *Glamour,* and running the beauty Web site eve.com; writing about style for publications like the *New York Times, Time,* and *More* magazine; and serving as a TV style expert for *Today, Oprah, CBS Early Show, Entertainment Tonight, Access Hollywood*, and others. But I wanted to take this book beyond my own experience, so I went out and interviewed every expert I knew—fashion stylists, beauty talents, shoe designers, bra specialists, retailers, cosmetic dentists, dermatologists, podiatrists, plastic surgeons, wardrobe advisers, eyewear pros, nutritionists, fitness gurus, etc.—to help me put together the ultimate master class on Hiding the Fat. Because we all need to have an easy-to-reference book on this subject sitting on our nightstands, right now.

Just as my first book, *How Not to Look Old*, helped women around the world learn fast and effortless ways not to look old, this is the essential book that pulls together all the latest information on what you need to do not to look fat.

The question that every woman I know asks herself before she walks out of the house is not, "Do I look chic?" or even, "Do I look good?" but rather, "Do I look fat?" Don't blame yourself for not knowing the answer. Obviously, a lot of us don't, because if we did, we wouldn't be walking around in the clothes we're currently walking around in. No woman *wants* to look fat or has said to herself at the time of purchase: "I realize that this dress will actually make me look ten pounds heavier, but I'm good with that." Every woman believes that she's making a wise buy. So how come we often get it so wrong?

The body-shape approach toward what to wear—forever discussed in style books, fashion magazines, and on TV style segments—isn't working. Many

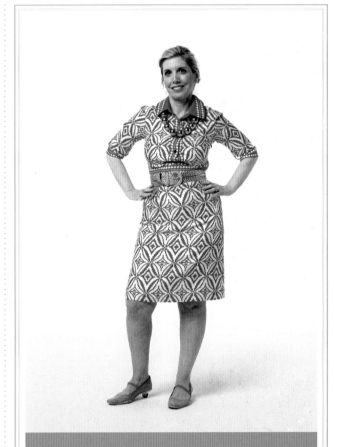

A HIGH-FAT LOOK

No, I'm not padded. This is how I look in a print that is just too busy for me—without shapewear, a super supportive bra, or heels. Plus, two heavy accessories is two too many. See my No Fat look on page 230, please!

women are still baffled by those body-shape paradigms—pear shape, apple shape, etc.—and have difficulty identifying with the model they're supposed to resemble because of all the variables: height, frame, muscle tone, age, where you live, what kind of work you do, and where you shop.

Nor am I a fan of those style books that try to reduce looking good to mathematical equations. Personally, I don't enjoy doing math. So please don't ask me to get out a tape measure and take my own measurements, then whip out a calculator and do a series of calculations to match them with a chart that determines my shape and fashion category.

And what about those style guides that ask us to identify with a celebrity and take her fashion cues? Oh, please! I'm not interested in channeling my inner Audrey or Jackie. Grown-up women don't feel the need to copy anyone else, be it a dead style icon or current Hollywood star. For me, the problem with so many of these style guides for women is that they're written by men. What I don't think many male style gurus realize is that most of us are proud of the women we have become. We are comfortable with who we are and what we have achieved; we love and appreciate our bodies for what they have done for us. It's just that our bodies sometimes don't reflect the real woman inside, for a whole host of reasons, some of which are beyond our control! We have strong opinions about fashion and know how we want to look. Maybe it's romantic one day, classic the next, boho the day after that. This is why I also don't go for style manuals that insist that we categorize our style personalities—sexy, preppie, ladylike—and stick with it; they don't allow us the freedom to be whoever we want to be on any given day.

As for books and magazines and TV shows predicated on looking good naked—they're unrealistic. While it would be a dream to look good without clothes, I think that's raising the bar too high. At this stage, I will happily settle for looking good dressed—the way I look in my normal everyday life. Are you with me?

That's why I've come up with a fast and simple way to determine whether a piece of clothing is going to pack on the pounds. It's the "No Fat Clothes" Diet. All you have to do is think about each piece of clothing in terms of how fattening it is for you. Assess whether a particular item is high fat or no fat. Simply steer clear of high-fat clothes, those guaranteed to make you look fatter than you are. Wear no fat as often as you can. How easy is that?

For speed, the first part of *How to* Never *Look Fat Again* is organized by body parts. You know what your personal issues are better than anyone else, so if you're time crunched, you can read about just that specific part. Or, if you only want to focus on how you look when you're at the gym or on special occasions, go to the chapters that zero in on tricky purchases such as swimwear, workout gear, and evening dresses.

My message in *How Not to Look Old,* where I talked about all the tricks I've learned to help you hide your age, was that it's not just a matter of vanity. Looking young is essential today to your personal survival in a competitive work world and a youth-obsessed culture. I feel exactly the same way about not looking fat. Just as looking old is a stigma in the workplace, so is showing the extra pounds. Even if we don't like it, that's the way it is.

It's not news that being overweight is a stumbling block to success in America and that overweight people are often subjected to discrimination at work. Ten years ago, Mark Roehling, then a professor of management in the business school at Western Michigan University, analyzed twenty-nine weight-loss studies in addition to his own and concluded that weight discrimination in the workplace is worse for women than men. "Women who are even slightly overweight suffer a wage penalty," Roehling said. "In contrast, men who are slightly overweight experience a wage bonus. They actually earn a little bit more." Weight discrimination, he concluded, is an acceptable bias in America, because people he spoke with didn't feel the need to hold back their anti-fat prejudices. ("Weight-Based Discrimination in Employment: Psychological and Legal Aspects," *Personnel Psychology,* 1999).

Employers can get away with such prejudices because, unlike other minority groups, overweight people aren't protected by anti-discrimination laws. "If you have three people applying for two jobs and they all have the same objective qualifications, but one is an ex-felon, one is an ex-mental patient, and one is overweight, the one person who won't get a job is the overweight person," Roehling said. Shocking, isn't it?

According to the Obesity Society, inequities for the overweight in "employment settings, health care facilities and educational institutions" were due to "widespread negative stereotypes that overweight and obese people are lazy, unmotivated, lacking in self-discipline, less competent, noncompliant and sloppy." In fact, weight discrimination was actually found to be more prevalent than race discrimination; it ranked third in discrimination, behind gender and age. ("Perceptions of Weight Discrimination: Prevalence and

As for books and magazines and TV shows predicated on looking good naked—they're unrealistic. While it would be a dream to look good without clothes, I think that's raising the bar too high. At this stage, I will happily settle for looking good dressed—the way I look in my normal everyday life. Are you with me?

Comparison to Race and Gender Discrimination in America." *International Journal of Obesity,* 2008).

In another study, participants were asked to rate normal-weight and obese job candidates on leadership potential, predicted success, likelihood of selection and starting salary. Normal-weight candidates scored 16 percent higher on the starting salary ranking, and were 14.7 percent more likely to be chosen as the right person for the job ("Do Antifat Attitudes Predict Antifat Behaviors?" *Obesity,* 2008) .

You'd think that with all the attention on weight in our culture, people would stop ordering those cheeseburgers with a side of fries, a milk shake, and apple pie. But the latest statistics show that the number of overweight Americans is growing—and the number of those actually obese is growing even faster. If you fall in that obese group—defined as people who are more than a hundred pounds overweight—you really

LET ME INTRODUCE YOU TO THE SPECIAL SECTIONS YOU'LL FIND SPRINKLED THROUGHOUT THE CHAPTERS OF THIS BOOK:

YOU KNOW YOU HAVE IT WHEN...

A checklist to see if you have the problem in question.

HIGH-FAT/NO-FAT LISTS

Clothing and accessories are analyzed for their potential fat-making content. These are the lists to take with you when you go shopping.

SWAP-OUTS

Newer ways to hide fat. How to exchange dated pieces for the current fashion solution, so that you look neither fat nor frumpy.

10 THINGS THAT MAKE YOU LOOK FAT

Tips that address the styling of outfits.

THINNER BY TONIGHT! INSTANT GRATIFICATION

Fierce, fast ways to drop a dress size in seconds.

DON'T WASTE A PENNY ON...

The bottom line on beauty bull and fashion hype.

IF YOU'RE PETITE...

Special call-outs for the majority of women in the United States, who are under five-foot-four.

IF YOU'RE SIZE 14 & UP...

Special call-outs for women who have been challenged to find cool clothes in their sizes.

GOING TO EXTREMES

Cosmetic surgery, dermatological treatments, and new-age solutions to body issue dilemmas. Even if you aren't in the market, you want to be in the loop about what's out there and whether it really works.

BRILLIANT BUYS

Specific recommendations for the products that really work—brands, style numbers, prices, retailers, and shopping Web sites.

VOWS

Promises to make to yourself to keep from dressing high fat.

DON'T YOU DARE...

Just one last thing that even your best friend might not tell you.

need to do something about it before you can get the full benefit of my book. Dr. Pamela Peeke—the fitness and nutri-shrink guru who tells it like it is in such books as *Fight Fat After Forty, Body for Life for Women, Fit to Live*—says that women who are more than fifty pounds overweight are especially in need of addressing the psychological issues underlying their excess weight. "At fifty pounds overweight, there are neon signs flashing," she explains.

But there's a big difference between being obese and simply being overweight—the category that most of us fall into. Although the slimming strategies in this book can be useful to everyone, they will have the most dramatic effect on women who are in the healthy weight range but still have a bit more they'd like to lose.

There was a time in my life when I was as much as thirty pounds overweight (you'll hear more about that on page 71). But even the extra pounds that I'm currently carrying around are getting harder and harder to take off. It's difficult to believe now, but I used to brag about my ability to lose weight fast. I would pop into a Weight Watchers meeting, have a quick weigh-in, limit myself to 18 points a day, work out a couple of times a week, and—voila!—the weight would always fall off. I felt very confident and in control knowing that I had this fail-safe method that I could always turn to whenever I went off-track. That plan now falls into the category of things I used to believe in that I can no longer rely on—like the stock market and my 401(k). The old tricks for shedding pounds just aren't working anymore. I'm sure I'm not the only woman who feels this way.

Over the past year, in my effort to lose those extra pounds, I tried the South Beach Diet. I re-upped at Weight Watchers, even registered for weightwatchers. com. I boosted my spinning classes from three days a week to six. I invested in a personal trainer for weight lifting. I bought all the hot new diet books. And as Oprah suggested on her show, I even had my thyroid checked. (Too much information, I'm sure, but yes, I did have an underactive thyroid. Unfortunately, taking medication to keep it in check did not help move the needle on my scale.) Nothing seemed to work.

Finally, my doctor told me that with menopause, women gain an average of six pounds. (I wish that was all that I gained!) Six pounds is perfectly normal; the weight just doesn't come off so easily anymore, and that's why women keep putting on pounds as they age. I don't know how I missed the e-mail about the need to cut back your calories and ramp up your exercise after menopause, but it probably went to spam along with the messages for acai berry cleanse, amazing diet tea, and lose weight with PomClear!

So I decided that I couldn't do this on my own any longer. I needed professional help. I went to see a nutritionist upon the urging of my friend Andrea Sachs, who was also an experienced Weight Watcher. Dietician and nutritionist Jennifer Andrus was the first to tell me that 18 points a day on Weight Watchers (my old benchmark) was too much food for me. Jen calculated the amount of calories I should consume per day to lose weight; I found out that I was taking in hundreds more calories a day than she figured I should be. What I've discovered is that I can't eat the same as I did ten years ago. No woman can.

The other thing I've learned in the past few months is . . . I don't have time for all this! At this particular moment in my crazy-busy life, with the reality of my

Why spend all that time and money going overboard to try to replicate the body of Malibu Fitness Barbie? There are so many other things you can do to shed those pounds—or to make it *appear* that you've shed them.

schedule, my deadlines, my travel, and my priorities, I simply can't indulge in an all-out, all-consuming body and weight-loss obsession. It would be nice to work out seven times a week, but these days I can barely manage three. I wish I could make healthy nutritious meals for breakfast, lunch, and dinner, but it's hard to find time to food shop, let alone cook. And I don't even have kids!

As I'm writing this, I'm reading in *W* magazine about the Tracy Anderson gym that is opening up in New York City's Tribeca. Tracy (who you'll be hearing from later, in chapter 14) is offering up the workout plan of her famous clients like Madonna and Gwyneth Paltrow to mere mortals like us. First, you have to get to her studio, then it's 90 minutes of a grueling workout a day, six days a week. The cost: about a thousand dollar initiation fee plus nine hundred dollar a month dues. She warned *W* editor Jamie Rosen that if you stop her program, your rear end (never mind your investment) will fall flat and back to its original position after two weeks. Plus there's a strict dietary component: gallons of green veggie juice, no dairy, no oil, brown rice is the devil, etc. Tracy says she's almost fully booked, but how many busy women in the real world can not only afford, but realistically commit to this? And for the rest of their lives?

Even if we had the time, money, and discipline of celebrities who make their living on the red car-

pet and whose cellulite is regularly hunted down by paparazzi to be front and center on magazine covers, is this what we really want to spend our time and our money doing? As evolved as women are right now, isn't it a throwback to be slaves to an unattainable, unsustainable, unrealistic body image? There is so much important work to be done on a global level and a personal level, isn't it just a little ridiculous to let the pursuit of the perfect body consume our lives?

Do we really need to have the thighs of Gwyneth? The arms of Madonna or Kelly Ripa? Jessica Simpson gained a few pounds, wore the wrong belt, and suddenly—hello!—she looked like every other American woman at Costco. But her weight gain was national news—the lead story on the entertainment shows, the cover of celebrity magazines, the front page of newspapers across the country. And Valerie Bertinelli? No one had seen her in years, but she became a hot commodity again by revealing her body on national TV (her bikini photos were one of *People* magazine's bestselling covers of the year) and was rewarded with her own syndicated TV show—all because she lost fifty pounds! Kirstie Alley, on the other hand, gained back all the weight she once so proudly lost—and her *Fat Actress* reality show is no longer a reality. She's onto her second show about weight called *Kirstie Alley's Big Life*. And, if you turn on the TV right now, you'll find at least ten shows about weight loss, from *The Biggest Loser* to *Ruby*.

With this book, I'm asking you to give yourself a break! Yes, you should diet. Yes, you should exercise. But you should also realize that even if you dedicated your days to making those few pounds go away, you probably still won't look as thin as the twentysomething super-skinny celebs who appear in the weekly tabloids and the sixteen-year-old models you see in fashion magazines. (For one thing, no one is airbrushing your rear end and thighs for any dimples of cellulite!) More important, you wouldn't necessarily be any healthier, either. I know what weight I can go up to and still, according to the physicians' charts, be considered healthy. I'm not going to go there, partly because I would have a closetful of clothes that I wouldn't be able to wear. But aside from that, I would just feel fat, not fit. For me to feel confident, happy, and well, I need to look and feel fit, not fat. That's the goal here.

My point is that if those few extra pounds aren't unhealthy but simply a matter of looking good—to yourself and to others—why beat yourself up over them? Throughout history, women have manipulated their bodies to conform to the fashionable shape of the time. Only in the last century has the ideal figure become, as Joan Rivers so aptly describes it, an ironing board with big boobs. Why spend all that time and money going overboard to try to replicate the body of Malibu Fitness Barbie? There are so many other things you can do to shed those pounds—or to make it *appear* that you've shed them. And now you have the book that tells you exactly what you need to do.

The bottom line? I don't have time for a body and weight-loss obsession. And probably, neither do you. Six pounds overweight? Twelve pounds overweight? I say, big deal. I'm not going to kill myself to get rid of them. I'm going to take the easy way out, and I'm inviting you to join me. Now, turn the page, and let's get you looking thinner by tonight! ●

Are Your Clothes Making You Look Fat?

IT'S NOT YOU; IT'S YOUR CLOTHES.

How else do you explain why on some days you look your thinnest and on other days, not so much—when you weigh exactly the same?

→There are high-fat clothes and no-fat clothes and those (low-fat) in-between. Most of us have all three categories—high fat, low fat, and no fat—hanging in our closets and filling our drawers.

As weight-conscious women, we are aware of calories as well as fat grams. We are constantly monitoring what we put in our mouths. If you have an entire pizza for dinner, you are not likely to top it off with a rich dessert. Because pizza alone is going to max out your calories and fat intake, pretty much no matter what diet you're on. Now if you stayed no-fat all day, when the dessert cart rolls up, you may feel like you can indulge in one perfect chocolate chip cookie. This daily internal negotiation that we have with food—"I'll eat this, I won't eat that"—is the same principle we need to apply to clothes: "I'll buy this, I won't buy that." Just like you wouldn't keep Mallomars in the kitchen if you were trying

to lose weight, you shouldn't store fattening choices in your closet if you want to look slim. Same concept.

Making strategic clothing choices for your specific body issues is the secret to dressing Fit Not Fat! Of course, you can (and should) diet and exercise, but neither of those are going to get you looking ten pounds thinner, ten years younger, and ten times sexier *by tonight.*

Here's how to look Fit Not Fat in a super-fattening big floral-print full skirt: Don't top it off with an equally fattening oversized white cotton blouson top with full sleeves. Instead, keep your top half (and everything else on your body) slim because you have maxed out your fat allowance with the skirt. So you choose a stretchy V-neck top that hugs your body and fabulously shows off your toned upper half—neck, shoulders, décolletage, waist, and arms.

You don't have a fabulous upper body to compensate for the super-fattening skirt? No problem—don't wear the skirt. Instead, go head to toe in a monochromatic dress or pants look. Which, as you will find out in the pages to come, doesn't have to be black and doesn't need to be boring.

Let's face it, stressing out about "What can I wear and not look fat?" consumes too much of our time— trying on clothes, looking in the mirror, figuring out if we look fat—and then we are forever returning our miscalculations.

You don't want to wear more than one piece of high-fat cloth-ing per outfit. Ideally, you want all your clothes to be zero fat. Fashion designers, stylists, tailors, and good personal shoppers all know what pieces make you look Fit Not Fat. Now you will, too, because in each chapter you'll find various pieces of clothing categorized into high-fat and no-fat lists. *Please note that the* *same piece can be high fat for one body issue and no fat for another. So no angry letters, please!* Once you have the list for your body issue, you will be able to assess how fattening that piece of clothing on the rack will be on your body, before you waste time bringing it into the dressing room. Why is this important? Of course, it's best if you can actually try everything on, but really, who has the time? If you can size up the fat factor in a nanosecond, you'll have more time to do all those other more important things in life. (And you'll look Fit Not Fat doing them, too.)

This book is dedicated to fast-tracking your "Do I look fat?" quandaries. Once we collectively nail this fat issue, we will move on with the self-assuredness of a woman who knows that she looks Fit Not Fat and therefore is in control. One great role model is Michelle Obama, who is not a size 2 but always looks strong and confident and pleased with herself, in whatever she wears.

Four basic ingredients pretty much determine whether a garment or accessory is fattening: shape, fabric, color, and fit. To assess the fat content of a piece of clothing or accessory in the abstract, we have to massively generalize. So please cut me some slack if you do indeed find a Pucci print puffer coat that makes you look ten pounds thinner!

Fit is the wild card here. Only you and your three-way mirror can figure it out. A good tailor can help ensure a great fit, but sometimes a tailor will convince you to salvage a piece that is simply not worth salvaging. (Just like a sales associate in a department store will tell you that something looks fabulous when you know it doesn't. It's called being on commission.) Reject a piece sooner rather than later, and you won't be throwing good money after bad. Here's to *not* having any more miscalculations, which are probably those clothes in your closet with the hangtags still on. ●

WILL IT MAKE YOU LOOK FAT?
HOW TO TELL

It's time to break the habit of wearing clothes that are better in theory ...
An outfit either creates a good impression of you or it doesn't.

LOOK AT THE SHAPE

HIGH-FAT pieces are oversized or have excessive amounts of fabric. As in, a super-sized boyfriend sweater, a sailor pant, a baby doll dress, a pleated skirt, a dirndl skirt, a balloon skirt, a fifties-style ball gown, a ruffled peasant skirt, overalls, harem pants, sweatpants, and an espadrille shoe that ties up on the leg. On the flip side, pieces that are too small to cover your frame leave too much exposed and are also high-fat. Stay clear of tube tops, hot pants, cut-off jeans, shorts suits, micro-minis, bikinis, bustiers, cutout dresses, and slit-up-to-there skirts, too.

LOW-FAT pieces provide coverage, but not much else. (I am not going to concentrate on this category of clothes in this book, as I assume you will want to look as slim as possible, but I'll explain this category here, so you can assess your current wardrobe.) Many of these are boring classics that just sit there on your body and don't particularly flatter it. Often, it's a tweed blazer, twin sweater set, a sweater dress, a mid-calf skirt, pants with side pockets, a denim jacket, loafers, flannel shirts, white shirts, cotton tees, or plain black pumps.

NO-FAT pieces are the hardest workers. Well-constructed shapers, they enhance your figure, create a svelte silhouette, hide the fat, and slurp you up in all the right places. They make you look better than you would look naked. Stock up on trim V-neck sweaters with three-quarter sleeves, a pencil skirt, boot-cut jeans, an A-line shift dress, a wrap dress, flat-front trousers, a full-coverage bra, a shapewear bike short, high-waist opaque stockings, a control camisole, a knee-length heeled boot, and a pair of nude high heels.

LOOK AT THE FABRIC

HIGH-FAT fabrics are, unfortunately, the most alluring, heavy on shine and texture. Be wary of wide-whale corduroy, crushed velvet, metallic, leather, patent leather, suede, down, mohair, angora, brocade, taffeta, bouclé, sequins, satin, beading, quilting, embroidery, tulle, fringe, flannel, terry cloth, toile, fur (real or faux), chiffon, horizontal stripes, and big prints—houndstooth, floral, plaids, Pucci-esque.

LOW-FAT fabrics are those that are comfortable and wearable but don't particularly go out of their way to enhance your shape. The most popular include cotton, denim, plain velvet, silk, lace, wool crepe, and wool gabardine.

NO-FAT fabrics have a little something extra that helps mold, shape, and hug your curves. You can't have enough jersey, cashmere, fine cotton, spandex, fine ribs, flat knits, matte crepe silk, wool rayon, or vertical pinstripes.

LOOK AT THE COLOR

HIGH FAT: neons, brights, primary colors, pastels, white.

LOW FAT: darker hues—navy, brown, charcoal, olive, burgundy, gray.

NO FAT: black, but a closetful of black clothes is so depressing. Try to limit your black purchases to anywhere you have body issues.

LOOK AT THE FIT

HIGH FAT: too big or too tight.

LOW FAT: passable, not amazing.

NO FAT: perfect fit—like it was made for you.

How do trends play into the fat equation? When I look at a fashion runway, I'm always rooting for those trends that I can wear without looking like a blob. I love a show if it has dresses, suits, jackets, and pants I will not look fat in. Military—yes! It's generally dark, slimming, and fitted. Safari—yes! Most women find smallish leopard prints flattering. Transparency—no! Not for those with serious flab. Pretty baby—no! Little girl dresses and puffed sleeves make everyone look pregnant. Honestly, most of the trends only look good on stick-thin models stalking the runway, teenage girls trolling the mall, or the twenty-something-year-old assistants at fashion magazines. You know that curating a personal style by what looks good on someone else leaves you with a closetful of pieces you don't feel good wearing. But once you start looking at the fat content of clothes, you'll be outing fat clothes on the spot. The goal is to become a very picky, or shall we say discerning, fashion editor. I know you can do this.

Here's the bottom line: If you have to ask the question "Does this make me look fat?" you already know the answer. But chances are, you're still tempted to wear the piece in question because of how you want it to look, because you love the designer, because you love the fabric or color, because of where you bought it, because it's on trend, because you paid too much for it, because, because, because.

Sorry, but we don't walk around with a letter of explanation pinned to our cropped jackets defending our choice of this garment. It's time to break the habit of wearing clothes that are better in theory—and see yourself in the same bright light that others see you. That outfit either creates a good impression of you or it doesn't. And, if it doesn't, summon up the courage to banish the offending garment to the giveaway bag.

What's lurking in your closet that's packing on the pounds? You'll have a better fix on those sartorial calorie-adding culprits after you take this quiz. ●

Here's the bottom line: If you have to ask the question, "Does this make me look fat?" you already know the answer.

THE "ARE YOUR CLOTHES MAKING YOU LOOK FAT?"
QUIZ

(1)
YOUR WINTER COAT IS

A. A metallic silver puffer that hits mid-calf

B. A short black puffer that's belted at the waist

C. A navy single-breasted wool or cashmere three-quarter-length coat

(2)
YOUR FAVORITE SKIRT IS

A. A denim mini

B. A boho-chic maxi

C. A black pencil that grazes the knees

(3)
MOST OF THE CLOTHES IN YOUR CLOSET ARE

A. Bright hues and bold patterns

B. Solid colors

C. Black

(4)
YOUR FABRIC OF CHOICE IS

A. Satin

B. Cashmere

C. Jersey

(5)
YOUR EVERYDAY SHOES ARE

A. Platform wedges

B. Kitten heels

C. Knee-high black suede boots with a heel

(6)
YOUR JEANS ARE

A. Skinny jeans that taper at the ankle

B. Five-pocket with straight legs

C. Dark denim boot cut with a bit of stretch

(7)
YOUR BLACK PANTS ARE

A. Relaxed fit with elastic waist

B. Wide legged with cuffs

C. Slim cut in a Lycra® blend

continued

(8)
YOUR WHITE PANTS ARE

A. High-waisted

B. Stretch cotton capris

C. Flat-front trousers

(12)
YOUR UNDERWEAR OF CHOICE IS

A. Cotton boy shorts

B. A barely there thong

C. A seamless bike short with control

(9)
YOUR WORKOUT OUTFIT IS

A. An oversized T-shirt and sweats

B. A Juicy Couture velour tracksuit

C. Yoga pants and a tank top

(13)
YOUR BRA IS A

A. Lacy black push-up bra

B. Comfy white T-shirt bra

C. Supportive, full-coverage nude

(10)
YOUR STOCKING DRAWER HAS MOSTLY

A. Patterned stockings and colored tights

B. Nude hose

C. Black tights

(14)
YOUR FAVORITE SHAPEWEAR PIECE IS

A. Camisole

B. Bike short

C. Body suit

(11)
YOUR SWIMSUIT IS

A. A bikini

B. A tankini

C. A solid color one-piece

(15)
TO BED, YOU WEAR

A. Boxers and an oversized T-shirt

B. Cotton nightgown

C. Tank top and pajama bottoms

IF YOU ANSWERED . . .

MOSTLY A'S: You may be up on the fashion trends, but unless you are built like Brazilian supermodel Gisele Bundchen (and if you are, please don't stand near me) you risk looking fatter and frumpier than you actually are because the colors, fabrics, textures, and shapes you gravitate to are super-fattening. Think of your closet as the equivalent of a high-fat fridge crammed with cake, cookies, chocolate sauce, and [insert your favorite forbidden food here]. You need to quit those high-caloric pieces, so you won't be tempted when getting dressed. Don't worry about what you wore in the past. You're in the fat-free zone now. Promise yourself: No more fat clothes. Once you go chapter by chapter, you'll see a huge difference—not only in how you look, but how you feel. You'll be happier with yourself for taking action and switching to no-fat clothes from this day forward.

MOSTLY B'S: Your closet is packed with solid low-fat choices, and you have the right idea about what looks right, but your look could be even sleeker if you traded some of those low-fat pieces for no-fat pieces. Sometimes you may be tempted by a dress, a sweater, or a skirt even though you intuitively know it's not going to do you 100 percent justice. Next time that happens while you're shopping, try a little self-control. Ask the sales associate to hold the piece in question while you shop around. In the next five minutes, picture yourself showing up at work or a party in that piece, looking ten pounds heavier than you actually are. Do you still want it? Summon up the willpower to tell yourself, and the sales associate, that it wasn't meant to be. Welcome to your first day of No-Fat Dressing. From now on, only buy no-fat. Once you see how much thinner you look, it won't be hard to say no next time.

MOSTLY C'S: Congrats! You're an extremely fashion-savvy woman whose closet is packed with lean, no-fat choices. You not only know what's hot, you know your bod—and what flatters it best. You probably look as thin as possible day in, day out. But if you still *feel* that you look fat, maybe there's something that's just a little bit off. Maybe you're not seeing yourself the way others see you. Then again, it could be the styling or the fit, but don't worry, we'll figure it out.

WITH THIS BOOK, YOU'RE ALL SIGNED UP FOR THE MASTER CLASS.

——

You'll discover how subtle little styling tricks can make you look thinner, taller, and sexier. From now on you'll be able to tweak your own outfits to perfection like a pro.

Who among us does not want to walk out of the house every day looking like we dropped a dress size or two? From now on, wear only no-fat clothes and you'll look Fit Not Fat every day, all year round, winter and even in summer, too.

Let's start at the top and work our way down.

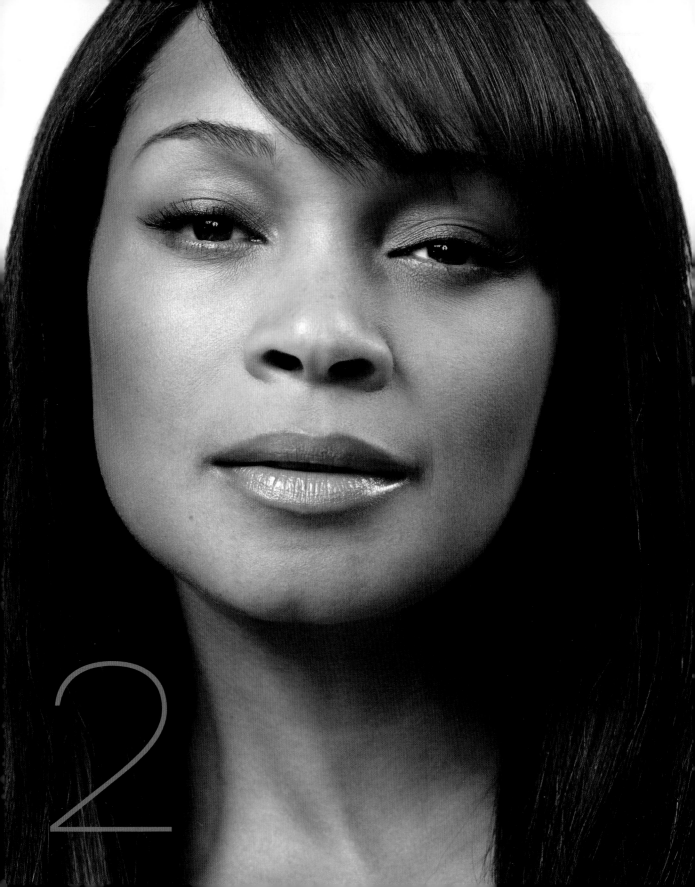

2

Wide Face

AKA

chipmunk cheeks, chubby cheeks, moon face, pumpkin face, pudgy punim, Humpty Dumpty

YOU KNOW YOU HAVE IT WHEN...
You haven't seen cheekbones since the Reagan administration . . . You can barely see your eyes when you smile . . . Photos make you look like you're storing away nuts for the winter . . . You have more than one chin.

→ When it comes to looking plump, a fat face is not the worst thing you can have. In fact, at this very moment, imagine the pileup of fashionable women cooling their Manolo Blahniks in doctors' reception rooms from New York to L.A., waiting to get fat injected *into* their faces to plump up their lips, cheeks, temples, smile lines, nasolabial folds, etc. Today having a fat face is preferable to having a long, drawn, thin, gaunt face, especially as you reach the higher ground of birthdays. But you don't want to appear roly-poly with multiple chins! No way! Not when the facial aesthetic of the moment is full, juicy, and heart shaped, with sculpted cheekbones and a clean jaw line. How do we know this?

Ask a plastic surgeon what women want. New York City's David Rosenberg, MD, PLLC, in demand for his more modern face-lifts, describes the most requested facial features at the moment as "a natural appearance of robustness on the apples of the cheek and a very defined jaw line. Whether it be natural or surgically created, a jaw line and neck complex that shows the underlying bone structure is very aesthetic. A chubby face," he says, "is unappealing because you can't see any architecture." So there you have it: Pudgy cheeks, a slack jaw line, and a blubbery shapelessness are what you don't want.

But are we all going to line up to see Dr. Rosenberg? Of course not. A fat face is not the reason to get a face-lift, and you don't want to resculpt your face so that you look like a completely different person. Do you? You just want to give yourself more definition by playing up or playing down certain facial features. The most talented hairdressers and makeup artists know how to fake the face of the moment to make you look more sculpted, baby! You've seen the photos of celebrities without makeup. When they're getting their Starbucks in the morning, they don't look any better than you or me. But in the hands of their glam squads, they are transformed and made to look positively chiseled, showing a little bone atop the cheeks and under the jaw line. How do they do it? By the end of this chapter, you'll know what they know. ●

for a Wide Face

→BECAUSE YOUR FACE IS A RELATIVELY small space, every feature must be considered and possibly tweaked to make you look slimmer, sexier, and more attractive. If it's not working for you, it's working against you. Is it your hair that's making you look fat? Your hair color? Makeup? Brows? Eyewear? Nose? Teeth? Let's take a look, feature by feature.

IS YOUR HAIR FATTENING?

Hair is your most powerful transformational tool. Style, length, texture, color, shine, volume, health . . . you want all these factors working in sync to up your attractiveness. Say you have a pretty good-looking face shape and not an excessive amount of facial width. If you frame it with high-fat hair, you're going to look fat. So you want to flaunt a mane that doesn't add inches to your face. Here are some strategies to get your hair and face to complement each other in the most slenderizing way possible.

IS YOUR HAIR COLOR MAKING YOU LOOK FAT?

Highlights or lowlights? Choose one or the other because the last thing you want is a single block of the same color covering your entire head. Brad Johns, one of the top hair colorists on the planet, lightens up the look of celebrities and real women (like me) at the Brad Johns Studio in the Red Door Spa at Elizabeth Arden in Manhattan. He offers up this advice to take to your colorist wherever you live: "Heavy hair is solid one-color hair. Whether you're a redhead, a brunette, or a blonde—if your hair is all the same shade, it's going to make you look heavy." If you love dark, dramatic hair and want a face that's long and lean, frame the face in shades of caramel highlights. If you're

> If you remember just one thing about hair, remember that your hair needs to be in proportion to the rest of you.

blonde and you want to narrow your face, frame it in bright, light-colored highlights—and add a few to the top, too. To give blonde hair natural-looking dimension, the hair underneath should be darker than what's on top, not the same exact blonde. Brad admits, "If someone has a round face, you need to do

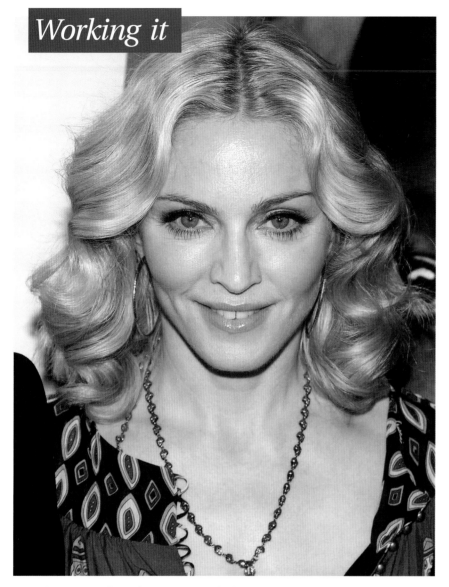

MADONNA — A face that's juicy and plumped in all the right places.

the time between visits by touching up your roots yourself with an at-home touch-up kit. Another way is to talk to your colorist about how best to minimize your beauty bill without sacrificing your look. He/she might have a less expensive way to create the magic, or an assistant wiling to follow instruction at a fraction of the cost!

PS: If you're younger and have the urge to put a pink streak in your hair, thinking that it will distract everyone's attention away from your size, don't. It always backfires and makes you look like you're trying too hard to be cool. The Manic Panic only works on Halloween or if you're still in high school.

IS YOUR HAIRSTYLE MAKING YOU LOOK FAT?

Unless you're playing Nikki Blonsky in a remake of *Hairspray,* big fat hair will only get you a "big hair, big girl" look.

If you remember just one thing about hair, remember that your hair needs to be in proportion to the rest of you. So don't do small hair if you have a big body, and don't do big hair on a small body. This is something that a lot of women get wrong. Just think about it: If you have a wide face, a super-short haircut can make your face and neck look even wider. But hair that's too long on a heavy face is not flattering, either; it's the equivalent

a little bit of magic with hair color." Unless you have a talent for hair color, this kind of magic is not something easily done solo at the bathroom sink with a box of home hair color. If you can splurge on just one beauty treatment done by

a professional, hair color is it. It's worth paying for that magic, the way your colorist can frame the face with various shades that will emphasize some features and deemphasize others. One way to get around the high cost of hair color is to extend

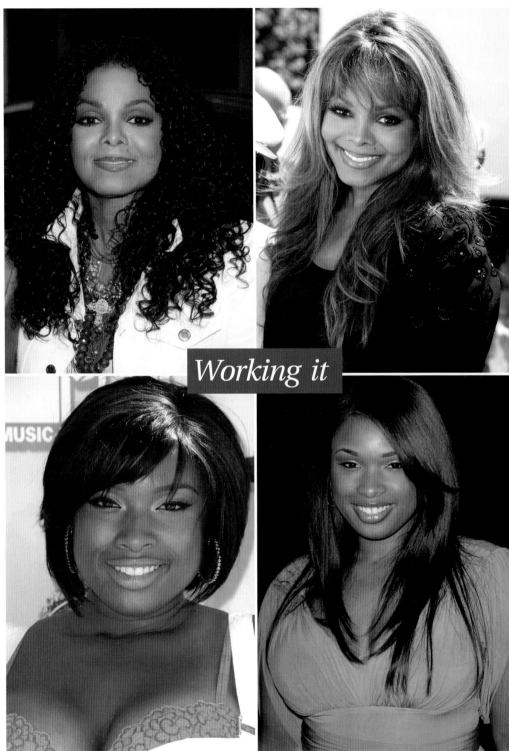

JANET JACKSON
Taking inches off the face with hair color and texture.

Working it

JENNIFER HUDSON
A severe blunt bob draws attention to a double chin. But longer hair with layers can be a beautiful distraction.

of having two heavy vertical lines on the sides of your face pulling you downward. Extremely long, straight hair that extends beyond the chest doesn't work because it can totally eliminate the neck—aka the squat mushroom effect.

Your best bet? One of the most universally flattering lengths is two to three inches below the collarbone because it brings the eye away from the widest part of the face, past the neck, down below the shoulders. Longish layers that curve around the neck are a sexy way to whittle width off, too. If you have a short, chunky neck but a strong jaw, you may look awesome with a medium-length choppy shag, shorter in front to flaunt the jaw line, longer in the back pieces to hug (and obscure) the neck.

What you don't want to do is get a blunt cut, ever again. Making a face appear less like a chipmunk and more like a swan is a matter of adding layers. Hairstylist Oscar Blandi, who has tousled the tresses on such glamorous stars as Jessica Biel and Jennifer Garner, at the Oscar Blandi Salon in New York City, advises, "Stay away from all one-length hair, because it's just a solid block that frames the face and neck, accentuating a double chin. If you have a heavier face, you don't have defined cheekbones, so you want a haircut that creates those concave angles for you." Sculpting the face

with framing layers is the solution. "The softer, more wispy and tousled, the better you're going to look," says Brad Johns. "And the more severe your haircut is, the heavier you're going to look." Buh-bye to those one-length bobs with blunt ends that can make a wide head look

Side-swept bangs are very flattering, while full blunt bangs will shorten and widen your face.

wider and out of proportion with the rest of the body. Blunt cuts are for the tall and skinny, like the iconic Anna Wintour.

Another strategic way to shave inches off your face is to hide some of it behind bangs, if your hair isn't curly or cowlicky. How they fall makes a huge difference. Side-swept bangs are preferable to full blunt bangs which will shorten and widen your face. "Low bangs plastered on your forehead are going to make you look heavy because it looks like your face is squeezing out of the hair," says Brad. Please do yourself a favor and don't cut your own bangs—they are way too critical to your look!

Brad Johns and Oscar Blandi are so expert at framing faces,

their tips for slimming facial features can be daunting. But if this list seems overwhelming, you don't have to change everything at once . . . instead, give yourself some time to digest and put some of these on your WIMP (When I'm Mentally Prepared) list! Here goes:

Ditch the middle part. It emphasizes the roundness of your face. Try a side part or high side part instead.

Don't be a stiff. Stiff hair is fat hair. Hair that moves freely backward, forward, and side to side is not. Swap high-hold sprays for soft-hold sprays. Choose soft gel over hard gel. No more heavy-duty sculpting wax or heavy-duty anything for that matter. Always start with just a tiny bit of product . . . you can always add more.

Control the frizz. Uncontrollable fluff is fattening. Use anti-frizz serums and shampoos and conditioners made specifically for frizzy hair types. The cool button on your dryer will lock the straightness in place. Blandi does a combo of hot then cold with each piece while blow-drying to set the style.

Don't be cutesy. No Heidi-like braids or any kind of pigtails. They only add width.

Don't be a flat head. Volumizing products will help provide a little lift to hair that's plastered to your face, which Brad refers to as the "cake-batter effect." As if someone were to dump cake batter on your head and the heavy mixture made your hair cling to your face and weigh you down. Very fattening indeed!

Lose the hair accessories that look as though they belong on a Christmas tree. We're talking the equivalent of wearing a holiday sweater in your hair—bells, green and red bows, reindeer headbands. When it comes to headbands, go thinner rather than thicker. Also don't engage more than one hair accessory at a time. And if something has claws—banana clips, etc.—toss it. Not only does it weigh you down, but it kills your look.

Go for the blow. There's nothing like an expert blowout to make you look and feel lighter. My mother and her generation still have weekly appointments at the "beauty shop" with their "beauty operators." If you have the time and the cash, it's not a bad idea to get blown out weekly. (There are women in Houston who see the hair guru Ceron three times a week!) In an ideal world, nicely priced quickie blowouts would be offered on every street corner and in every mall, but until they are, you might want to take a lesson from your stylist on how to blow it out yourself. To guarantee best results, invest in a professional quality blow-dryer and buy the exact same styling products they use at the salon.

IS THINNING HAIR MAKING YOU LOOK FAT?

If you are among those women who can slim down a round face with the right cut and color, consider yourself fortunate. Growing numbers of us don't have the luxury of hiding behind that security blanket. Some can now see patches of their bare scalps, no thanks to menopause; others lose their hair with chemotherapy. This is tough stuff to deal with, and it certainly puts the fat issue into perspective. But the good news is that there are more courses of action for women experiencing hair loss beyond getting a good wig. Eric S. Schweiger, MD, FAAD, a dermatologist who specializes in the treatment of hair loss for women at the Bernstein Medical Center for Hair Restoration in Manhattan, recommends the following:

See a doctor if your hair is not as full as it was once, because there might be other medical reasons at play.

Ask a doctor if a prescription for Rogaine is right for you. The generic version is Minoxidil and "women's strength" is 2 percent. You could see results in six months.

Fake it with Toppik (toppik .com). Like makeup for your scalp, these protein fiber particles cover and color bare scalp, making your hair look thicker. It's the secret weapon of many balding TV personalities!

Consider a hair transplant. "Thinning scalp hair, especially along the frontal hairline and top of the scalp, can definitely contribute to a patient looking heavier," says Dr. Schweiger. "After hair transplants, patients often are told by friends and family that they look younger, healthier, and thinner. Redistributing hair to the front has the effect of squaring off and framing the face to make it appear less round, creating the illusion of a thinner face." This surgery is definitely not just for men anymore.

ARE YOUR BROWS MAKING YOU LOOK FAT?

Skinny brows won't make you look skinny—in fact, they'll do just the opposite, make you look fat. "Thin brows make a heavy face seem even heavier," says Eugenia Weston, brow star of Beverly Hills, founder of Senna Cosmetics, and favorite makeup artist of Bette Midler, Sela Ward, and Ashlee Simpson. "A thicker brow makes a fuller face appear thinner and more proportioned, because it helps fill in all the open areas of a heavier face." If you have a large, round face, you are committing a major sin by skimping out on your brows. A pencil-thin line is not for you as you want a very soft, full arch with a longer tail at the outer edge.

How to get that full brow if your brow hairs are few and far between? New York dermatologist Debra Jaliman prescribes Men's Rogaine and tells her patients to apply a cotton tip of it to the brows once a day, to see new growth in three months.

One size does not fit all when it comes to brows, because they always need to be in proportion to the size of your face, your other features, and your facial architecture. A small face will be overwhelmed by a heavy brow.

There's a big payoff here if you get the brow right: You will be rewarded with an instant lift, which is why brows are sometimes called "the fifteen minute face-lift." A brow done well starts directly above your tear ducts, and the peak of the arch should line up with the outer edge of the colored iris at the three o'clock position. A shortcut to the well-shaped brow is Senna's Form-a-Brow stencil kit, which Eugenia created and which I have been using since I learned about it as *Glamour*'s beauty director. Imitators abound, but in all these years, none have bested it.

If you don't need to watch your beauty bill, leave your arches in the hands of a pro! Make an appointment with the best brow artist in town. PS: Your eyebrow color should always be a shade darker than your hair color.

IS YOUR EYEWEAR MAKING YOU LOOK FAT?

With a fuller face shape, you want a frame that makes your face seem longer and thinner. Circle frames are the trend of the moment, but who needs them? Perfect rounds and squares will only exaggerate a plump mug. If you have a round face, you need a slightly angled-upward rectangular frame. Why? Because "softer, angled-up edges give you an instant face-lift," says Eden Wexler, spokeswoman for Safilo USA, whose luxe designer eyewear brands include Marc Jacobs, Gucci, and Dior. →*continued on page 28*

SWAP–OUTS:
FRESHER WAYS TO LOOK LEAN AND SCULPTED

Instead of	→	Choose
Blunt bob		Layered bob
Circular eyewear		Rectangular eyewear
Hair up		Hair down
Heavy frames		Contact lenses
Flat hair		Volumized hair
Middle part		Side part
No bangs		Side-swept bangs
Round collars		V-necks
Severe cut		Soft layers

HIGH FAT *vs.* NO FAT

→ Subtle changes have a dramatic impact when your canvas is this small. Starting with your hair, try a side part rather than a straight down the middle one. Cut long, wispy bangs and you'll hide an expanse of forehead. Pump up the volume with styling product. Grow out a chin-length bob or fake it with hair extensions. (Really, who can even tell?)

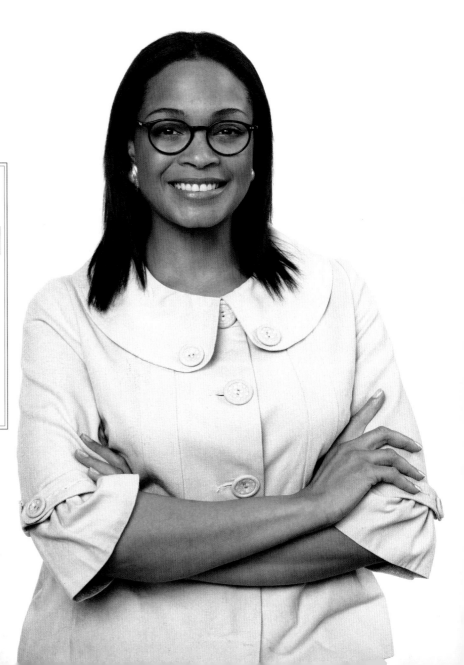

WORST FAT-FACE OFFENDERS

HIGH FAT
× Bare forehead
× Flat hair
× Middle part
× Rounded eyewear
× Severe bobs

HIGH FAT:
The circular specs, large button earrings, and round collar neckline are proof positive that wide circles contribute to an overall chunkiness, accentuating a plump face.

BEST BET
FACE THINNERS

NO FAT

√ Hair with body

√ Light, bright highlights around the face

√ Shaped, groomed brows

√ White, strong, vertical teeth

√ Wispy bangs

NO FAT:
Eye-grazing bangs, longish layered hair with lift, vertical earrings, a V-neck sweater, extended eyeliner, flirty faux lashes, and contoured cheekbones . . . a sexy, sculpted look.

When it comes to fit, you don't want frames that come up too high over the brows or too low, where they are resting on your cheeks. "On a round face, some wider glasses wrap around and hug the face, which is not desirable," says Eden. As for color, dark heavy frames and all those crazy brights and loud animal prints can be fattening.

IS YOUR MAKEUP MAKING YOU LOOK FAT?

If you can't remember the last time you had a makeup lesson from a pro, take an hour out of your life to change it. You may need a makeup face-lift. Find the best makeup artist in town, plunk yourself at the

Below, you'll find directions that will take the weight off your face and make you look thinner, lighter, softer, more radiant, and sexier!

counter, and take notes. The dirty little secret of the beauty biz is that technique is just as important as product. You can ring up your credit card and purchase every single Brilliant Buy in the book, but if you don't know what to do with it once

you get home, what's the point?

Below, you'll find directions that will take the weight off your face and make you look thinner, lighter, softer, more radiant, and sexier! I know that there are those of you who can't bear reading through directions of any kind, whether it's your iPhone, GPS, exercise, or makeup. Same here. So take this book to the counter, show it to the pro, and let him or her demo the techniques for you on one half of your face while you do the other. Unless you're really great with a brush, trust me, it's the only way.

Let me introduce you to two of the most talented makeup pros in the business. I had the amazing Stella Mikhail, who did my makeup for my most recent appearance on *Oprah,* meet me at the Laura Mercier counter at Neiman Marcus in Northbrook Court the last time I was in Chicago. If you live in the area, book her! It's not easy to hire star makeup artist Mally Roncal, who has her own line of makeup, as she's often making up Beyoncé and Jennifer Lopez and appears as part of the Tyra show's glam squad, which is where we did some makeovers together. But now you're going to learn how to make your face look thinner from the best.

GET RID OF EYE PUFFINESS

Puffy pockets under the eyes and droopy, overhanging lids can make

you look fat. First, let's deal with the fat pads. Before you start the makeup, you need to reduce the puffiness (and conceal any crinkles) with a hydrating eye cream. Every makeup artist has a favorite, and it doesn't have to be pricey. Stella loves Natura Bissé Diamond Drops and Laura Mercier's Flawless Skin Eye Serum. For special occasions, Stella applies an eye treatment (Natura Bissé Ice-Lift) on top of the eye cream for enhanced moisturizing. Next she paints Laura Mercier's Secret Brightener under the eye area to bounce light off the dark shadows. She follows this with concealer—either Laura Mercier's or Clé de Peau's. "Layering concealer is important," she says. "You have to start really high up on the inner corners of the eyes where the eye meets the bridge of the nose." She paints the concealer on with a thin concealer brush, so it's evenly layered. She then smoothes it in with a damp sponge. "Mist your makeup sponge with a water bottle and blend down toward your cheek. Water helps the product hug the skin. Don't use a dry sponge or a dry finger—it will pucker the concealer up. And it won't look like skin anymore."

For puffy lids, de-puff first with soothing cucumber, chamomile tea bags, or a gel-based eye cream (again, Stella likes Natura Bissé Ice-Lift). After you bring the puffiness down, apply an eye shadow base that will hold and grab the shadow you're about to put on your lid. (I love the eye shadow bases from Laura Mercier and Trish McEvoy . . . they cover up discoloration and feel cool on lids.) Then, you're ready for shadow. "Start with a light neutral shadow and pat it in with an angle brush from your lash line to your brow bone. Then, with the angle brush, use a very deep shade of brown or gray and pat that on the lid. Finish by using a soft medium shade in the crease to contour and lift," Stella says. Another trick of hers is the signature Laura Mercier tight eyeline, where you line the root of the upper lash under the lid so that it creates a dark band at the lash line, making lashes look fuller—and false. She then lines the eye with a straightedge brush and cake liner that's water activated in blue, black, or brown. Don't just wet a shadow and use as liner, she warns. It will flake into the eye. Curl your lashes. Apply mascara and your eyes are good to go.

THE MAGIC OF HIGHLIGHTING

The modern way to minimize a full-moon face is by highlighting. "Gone are the days we would use brown or taupe eye shadow for contouring," says Mally Roncal. "The number-one trick to thinning out your face is highlighting." To make smile lines disappear, Roncal first applies a primer all over the face. Then, she dabs a creamy concealer in the crease of the lines. "The deeper your laugh lines, the more the cheek around them looks full," she says. If you highlight the laugh lines, the lines look pulled forward." It's a way of diminishing them and making them look less pronounced. Roncal uses skin-toned powder and softly brushes it on the cheekbone, hairline, chin, and cupid's bow of the lip to finish.

CREATE ANGLES WHERE THERE ARE NONE

If your nose has extra pudge or is missing a defined bridge, no one has to know it. Makeup artist Stella Mikhail creates a more angular face by contouring, with three different shades of highly pigmented stick foundation (she likes Laura Mercier's) and blending them with a damp makeup sponge. "If you don't have a bone on the bridge of your nose, for example, then you have to create one," she says. Here is how she shades the bridge of the nose with stick foundation.

1) All over your face, use the middle shade of stick foundation, and blend to perfection with a makeup sponge.

2) Then pick up the lightest shade of the three foundations (it should be a shade or two lighter than the one you would wear all over your face) and draw a vertical line down the center of the nose, and then with the same shade, draw lines under each eye.

3) Using the darkest of the stick foundations, draw a vertical line on each side of the nose. "This thins out the nose and makes the nose and the nostrils look slender," she says.

4) If your nose has a too-wide tip, draw a line with the darker stick foundation across the tip of the nose and the nostrils. Remember, darker always makes lines recede, while lighter highlights them and brings them forward.

5) Your face should now look like war paint, so carefully blend all lines with a makeup sponge, but not so much that it all comes off!

GET RID OF A DOUBLE CHIN

Stella's same contouring sticks can help minimize the look of a double chin. Take the darkest shade of foundation, and apply it at the edge of the chin bone, working your way down the neck, blending over the double chin. After blending the product in with a makeup sponge, she sweeps it all over the chin area with a pressed powder in matte bronze (from Laura Mercier) to blend. ●

Thinner by Tonight!

INSTANT GRATIFICATION

Pull your hair into a high ponytail then lightly tease at crown. It will bring out your bone structure and make your face look leaner.

Dust your T-zone with compressed translucent powder to cut down any shine.

Shape your brows. Use a stencil kit to make it goof-proof.

Apply a plumping lip gloss in a shade of pink.

Get sleek with a blowout or give yourself one.

Do the blush face-lift. Apply pink or peach cream blush about an inch under the middle of the eye. Blend it out so it spreads over the tops of the apples of your cheeks. It pulls everything up!

Switch your eyewear to a light-colored plastic frame, in a rectangular shape.

Going to Extremes: *Facial Features*

TEETH. If you think that I'm going tell you that the shape of your teeth can make a difference in how your face looks, well, I don't want to hold out on you! Remember that every facial feature has the potential to either add or subtract visual inches. "By manipulating the shape and position of the teeth, you can actually make the face look narrower," says New York cosmetic dentist Jeff Golub-Evans, DDS, who designs smiles on famous faces. Back in the '80s, supermodels seeking a heart-shaped face (high cheekbones on top of sunken, hollowed-out cheeks) actually asked their dentists to yank out their upper back molars! There's a kinder, gentler way to achieve that same lean look today. Dr. Golub-Evans reveals that he "angles inward" the upper back upper molars using clear braces like Invisalign (which still falls under the category Extreme).

NOSE. Next time you look at celebrity transformation photos, zoom in on the nose. Getting a nose job is common in Hollywood circles; getting a good one, for some reason, is not. Whether the nose in question is humpy, wide, or bulbous, traditional rhinoplasty was the fourth most popular cosmetic plastic surgery in 2008 with 152,434 served, according to the American Society for Aesthetic Plastic Surgery.

Because your nose sits in the middle of your face, if it is too big, too bumpy, too wide, or too fat, everyone takes notice. If your nose becomes a nonissue, the eye goes elsewhere. A pretty nose can set the agenda for the face—as in, slender nose, slender face. But you might be interested in the newer ways to get a better-looking nose. The non-surgical nose job uses an injectible filler, such as Restylane or Radiesse, to reshape the nose

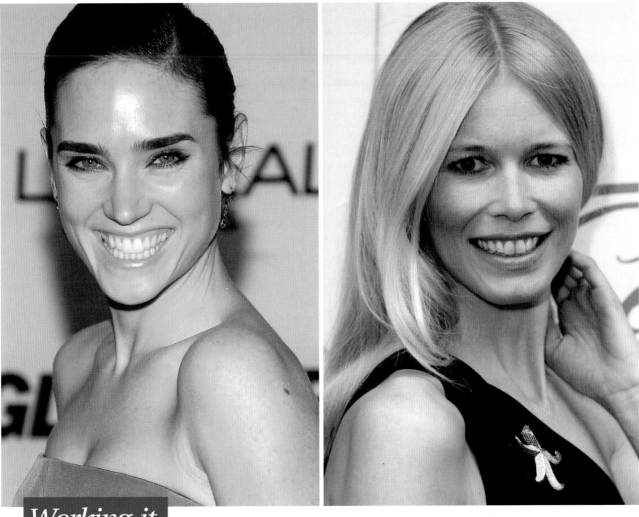

Working it   Long, lean, toothy smiles . . . only their dentists know for sure.
JENNIFER CONNELLY, CLAUDIA SCHIFFER

and even out the profile. This fifteen-minute nose job, as it's referred to, does not solve the problem of too large a nose, only nasal abnormalities such as bumps and bulges. Downside: It only lasts as long as the filler lasts, so you would need to redo in eight months or so. The cost over time may not be worth it.

For a bulbous nose, instead of traditional rhinoplasty in which the bone is broken, Dr. Rosenberg nips the tip and cuts the fat out. "I hear the words 'the tip of my nose is fat' all the time," he says. "A defined nasal tip is angular and gives the impression that the rest of the face has more structure." He narrows the base of the nose by stitching the two pieces of cartilage closer together. "The face looks considerably thinner after surgery," he says. No swelling and bruising makes this a more appealing option than rhinoplasty as usual. ●

BRILLIANT BUYS

EYES

EYELINER

Sonia Kashuk Dramatically Defining Long Wear Gel Liner, $8.99; Target.

Estée Lauder Double Wear Stay-In-Place Eye Pencil, $19; Macy's, esteelauder.com.

Neutrogena Nourishing Eyeliner, $8.49; mass retailers, drugstore.com.

Laura Mercier Eye Liner, $22; Sephora, lauramercier.com.

Maybelline New York Lasting Drama gel liner, $9.99; mass retailers, drugstore.com.

L'Oréal Paris Extra-Intense Liquid Pencil Eyeliner, $8.49; mass retailers, drugstore.com.

EYE SHADOW BASE

Smashbox Photo Finish Lid Primer, $20; Sephora.

Laura Mercier Eye Basics, $24; Bloomingdale's, lauramercier.com.

BeneFit Cosmetics Stay Don't Stray, $24; Sephora.

Trish McEvoy Eye Base Essentials, $25; trishmcevoy.com.

MASCARA

Yves Saint Laurent Mascara Volume Effet Faux Cils, $30; Sephora.

Dior Diorshow Unlimited, $24; Bloomingdale's, sephora.com.

Lancôme Hypnôse Mascara, $24.50; Bloomingdale's, sephora.com.

EYELASH CURLER

Laura Mercier Eyelash Curler, $16; lauramercier.com.

EYE MAKEUP REMOVER

Visine Total Eye Soothing Wipes, $5.99; drugstore.com.

HAIR

Aveeno Active Naturals Nourish + Condition Leave-In Treatment, $6.49; mass retailers, drugstore.com.

L'Oréal Paris EverPure Sulfate-Free Color Care Moisture Shampoo, $6.99; mass retailers, drugstore.com.

Garnier Fructis 3-Minute Undo Dryness Reversal Treatment, $5.99; mass retailers, drugstore.com.

Living Proof Full Thickening Cream, $14; sephora.com.

Kerastase Resistance Ciment Thermique Heat-Activated Reconstructor Milk for Weakened Hair, $36; drugstore.com.

LIPS

Maybelline New York Color Sensational Lipcolor in 005 Pink Sand and 045 Pink Me Up, $7.49; CVS/pharmacy.

Neutrogena MoistureShine Lipstick SPF 20 in 200, Anything Rose, $9.49; mass retailers, drugstore.com.

Guerlain Rouge G de Guerlain in Gemma 64, $46; Saks Fifth Avenue, sephora.com. In an elegant silver case.

Laura Mercier Crème Lip Colour in Rose, $22; Bloomingdale's, lauramercier.com.

Laura Mercier Shimmer Lip Colour in Pink Mist, $22; Bloomingdale's, lauramercier.com.

Sonia Kashuk Velvety Matte Lip Crayon in Pinky Nude, $7.99; target.com.

Dior Sérum De Rouge Luminous Color Lip Treatment, Dior SPF 20 in Radiant Pink 560 and Pearly Pink 470, $32; sephora.com.

SKIN

BLUSH/BRONZER

Sonia Kashuk Super Sheer Liquid Tint, $9.99; Target.

Topshop Makeup cream blush in Nutmeg, $12; Topshop, topshop.com.

BeneFit Cosmetics Coralista, powder blush, $28; Bloomingdale's, sephora.com.

CoverGirl & Olay Simply Ageless Sculpting Blush, $10.99; mass retailers.

CONCEALER

CoverGirl & Olay Simply Ageless Eye Concealer, $10.99; mass retailers.

Neutrogena Mineral Sheers Concealer, SPF 20, $13.99; mass retailers.

Laura Mercier Secret Concealer, $22; Bloomingdale's, lauramercier.com.

FOUNDATION

Maybelline New York Dream Liquid Mousse Foundation, $9.79; CVS/pharmacy, drugstore.com.

Giorgio Armani Luminous Silk Foundation, $59; Saks Fifth Avenue, giorgioarmanibeauty-usa.com.

CoverGirl & Olay Simply Ageless Foundation SPF 22, $13.99; mass retailers.

PRIMER

CoverGirl & Olay Simply Ageless Serum Primer, $13.99; mass retailers, drugstore.com.

L'Oréal Paris Studio Secrets Professional Magic Perfecting Base, $12.95; mass retailers.

Smashbox Photo Finish Foundation Primer UVA/UVB SPF 15 or Photo Finish Bronzing, $42; smashbox.com.

TINTED MOISTURIZER

Dior Hydra Life Pro-Youth Skin Tint SPF 20, $39; sephora.com.

Sephora Perfecting Tinted Moisturizer SPF 20 Oil-Free, $21; sephora.com.

Olay Definity Color Recapture, $24.99; mass retailers.

Top Shop Skin Tint, $20; topshop.com.

SKIN CARE

SPECIAL SKIN TREATS

Olay Professional Pro-X Intensive Firming Treatment Kit, $62; mass retailers.

DDF Revolve 400X Micro-Polishing System, $95; Sephora, ddfskincare.com.

DAY

Aveeno Ageless Vitality Elasticity Recharging System, $39.99; mass retailers, drugstore.com.

Olay Regenerist Micro-Sculpting Serum, $24.99; mass retailers, olay.com.

Elizabeth Arden Prevage Face Advanced Anti-aging Serum, $155; Bloomingdale's, sephora.com.

NIGHT

Philosophy Miracle Work Miraculous Anti-aging Retinoid Pads and Solution, $70; Sephora.

Patricia Wexler M.D. Dermatology Intensive Deep Wrinkle Treatment with MMPi-20 and Retinol, $60; Bath & Body Works.

Estée Lauder Advanced Night Repair Synchronized Recovery Complex, $47.50; Bloomingdale's.

DON'T WASTE A PENNY ON ...

Expensive, high-tech facials that promise instant face-lifts, plumping, or skin tightening. Galvanic facials, oxygen facials, electro-stimulating facials—call them whatever you want, but there is no science that proves that they can deliver the same results or even similar results as a dermatologist or plastic surgeon. The words "without injections" and "without surgery" are all we seem to hear. We want to believe that a series of facials can do more than just cleanse, exfoliate, extract blackheads, and pamper, but don't let anyone tell you that the results of a facial will last just as long as Botox or your average facial filler. Or that you need a series of these expensive facials and that there is a cumulative effect.

Look, massaging the skin manually will cause minor swelling, and stimulating the facial muscles underneath will give you a lift for a day or two. But do the math. Biting the bullet and going to a dermatologist for wrinkle removal and exfoliation (doctors administer higher dose glycolic peels) will probably be more cost effective, less time-consuming, and deliver more tangible results. Some fillers last up to nine months.

There are plenty of reasons to book a facial, if you have a big event such as a wedding or a reunion and want that extra glow, it's a delicious splurge. But the glow doesn't last very long.

Vows *for the* Face

- ☐ **I WILL NOT** part my hair in the center.

- ☐ **I WILL NOT** dye my hair black.

- ☐ **I WILL NOT** wear lipstick that is darker than my natural lip color.

- ☐ **I WILL** control my frizz with hair serum.

- ☐ **I WILL NOT** wear John Lennon–style round eyewear.

- ☐ **I WILL NOT** take a scissors to my own bangs.

- ☐ **I WILL NOT** wear hoop earrings the size of bracelets.

- ☐ **I WILL NOT** wear a thick headband or anything in my hair that has teeth, claws, or looks like it belongs on a Christmas tree.

- ☐ **I WILL NOT** get a perm.

DON'T YOU DARE...
Over-tweeze your brows.

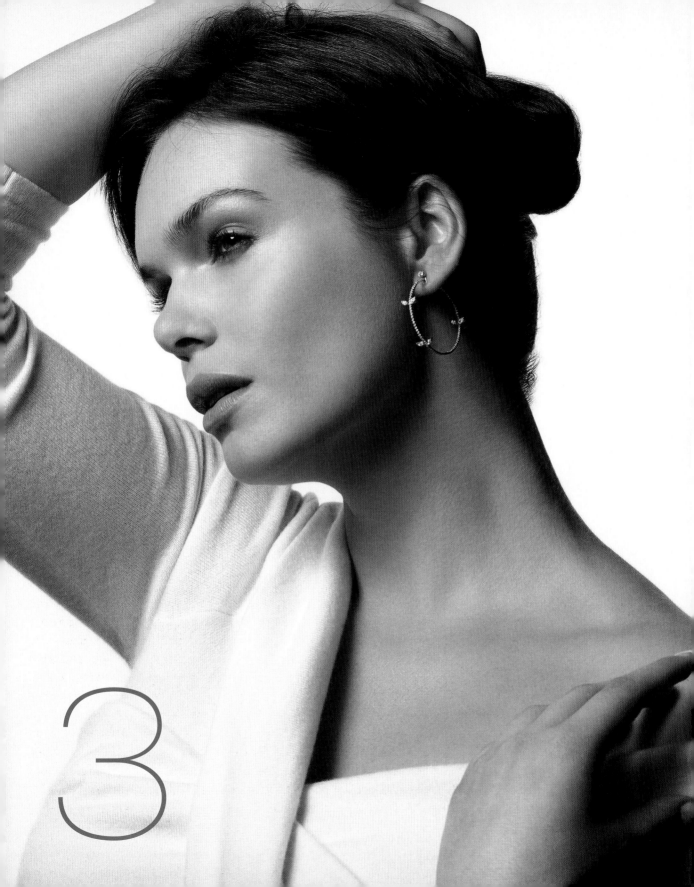

Thick Neck + Broad Shoulders

AKA
swimmer's
shoulders,
NFL shoulders,
bulldog neck,
no-neck,
hulk-neck,
fire-hydrant
neck, fat neck

YOU KNOW YOU HAVE IT WHEN...
Choker necklaces choke . . . You look like you're wearing shoulder pads when you're not . . . Sharp, structured shouldered jackets make you look ready for takeoff . . . . Your neck and face are about the same width . . . Your chin knocks your chest when you nod yes . . . A collarbone necklace fits like a choker . . . Necks on most turtlenecks are too long.

→ If you want to know what's happening in fashion right now, look to the White House. Today, more American women take their fashion cues from Michelle Obama than Agyness Deyn, Gemma Ward, or any of the hot models strutting the world's runways. The tipping point for the one-shoulder dress? Before Kate Winslet and Marisa Tomei at the Oscars, it was Michelle Obama at the Inaugural Ball in her beaded and appliquéd winter white gown by Jason Wu that inspired big-shouldered women to confidently expose those shoulders. The First Lady has ushered in a fresh way of looking at the female body, one that recognizes athletic, toned shoulders and arms as a source of strength and pride and as a new empowerment zone. Her bare shoulders seem to be sending the message, "I take time out for myself to work on my body, and you don't mess with shoulders like these."

If you, too, possess "swimmer's shoulders," as they were once called, the modern way is not to hide them but to flaunt them, making the statement that you're healthy, fit, and confident. Another reason to embrace strong shoulders is that they help balance out wide hips. If that is also a concern, having your upper and lower halves in proportion helps create that va-va-va-voom hourglass shape. However, if your shoulders are big, broad, but not exactly toned like Michelle's, you may feel more comfortable dodging high-fat details that add padding where you don't need it. You'll find those details later in this chapter.

And if you feel bad about your neck, don't, because you can fake a longer, more elegant neck, even if yours is short, wide, and sits on your shoulders like a bobble-head doll's. By making no-fat fashion choices, you can optically stretch your neck to look more Penelope Cruz, less Incredible Hulk. Creating a neck where there wasn't one, you'll also be gaining an erogenous zone . . . ideal for kissing, dabbing a divine fragrance, and hanging fabulous jewelry. You may know that a short, wide neck—like short wide legs, fat ankles, and stubby hands—is genetic, but it's not worth assigning blame, not when you can just as easily pick up tricks to dress around it. And, if a thick neck is not your issue, but a turkey neck is, some of the same strategies suggested here will apply. ●

for a Thick Neck + Broad Shoulders

FOR NECKS

→THE CONCEPT IS SIMPLE: the longer the neck, the thinner you look. So, if you have a short, wide neck, your mission is to do everything possible to create the illusion of more length from chin to chest. (Not a lot of room to work with, for sure.) You want to open up the area with necklines that dip below the collarbone, so skip necklines that close you in. The more skin displayed between chin and chest, the more elegant your proportions will appear—no matter what else is going on below. The road to an elongated neck starts with the neckline you need to wear from this day forward: the deep V.

Living in V-necks will simplify your life and make it easier for you to look your best, fast. The downward diamond optically elongates and narrows so you don't have a cutoff point where the actual neck stops, which gives the illusion of extra inches. You can collect V's in everything—camisoles, tanks, tees, sweaters, cardigans, dresses, and jackets. From shallow little mid-chest V's to deep just-above-the-bra dips, V's make

sleeveless dresses, as well as wrap tops or dresses, flattering. Stop short of showing cleavage crack, as that just looks trashy. Look for bras that dip low in front so you don't have to be checking to see if your bra is showing. Modify V's that are too low by sliding a V camisole just a hint higher beneath. Unbutton shirts, shirtdresses, blouses, polos, and henleys and spread the necklines open to form a V. After the V, your next best necklines are scoops and some cowls because they, too, will reveal your nice neck zone.

Relinquishing the turtle is imperative to have this nice expanse of skin showing. Women love to hide out in them, but slip on a turtle and your neck disappears. Remember the movie *Something's Gotta Give* in which Jack Nicholson's character teased Diane Keaton's about her penchant for wearing turtlenecks even in the heat of summer? She ultimately realized the error of her ways, and by the end of the movie, she was wearing V-necks and showing a sexy stretch of skin at the throat. If only getting a guy as appealing as Jack Nicholson in your sixties were that easy! It's certainly worth a try.

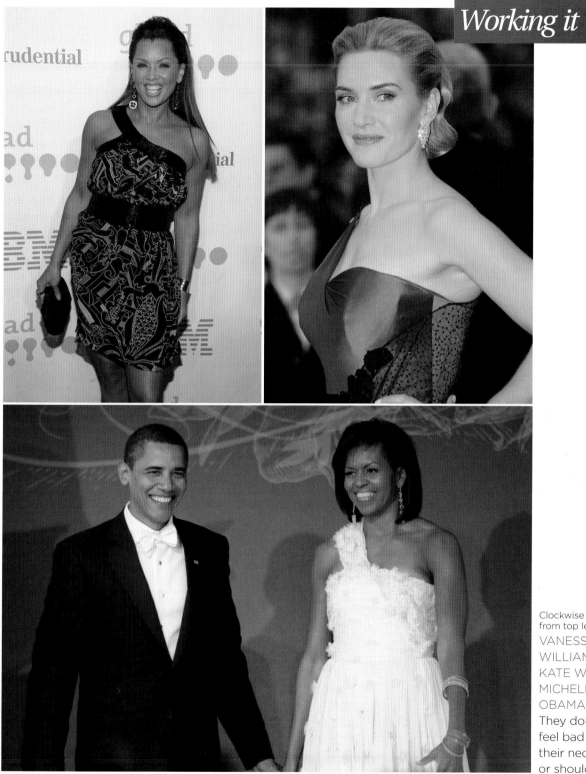

Clockwise
from top left:
VANESSA
WILLIAMS,
KATE WINSLET,
MICHELLE
OBAMA
They don't
feel bad about
their necks—
or shoulders.

FOR SHOULDERS

You've lucked out. The Fashion Gods are with you; we're experiencing a strong shoulder season. Women with substantial shoulders are flaunting them; women with smaller shoulders are wearing sculptural shoulder-padded jackets and dresses to ramp them up. If your shoulders are big, broad, and toned, bare them in halter necklines, strappy necklines, asymmetrical one-shoulder tops, and strapless gowns. (The diagonal of the one strap will cut a more flattering and provocative line than a full-on horizontal strapless gown.) If your shoulders are big, broad, and flabby, you can conceal them in capes, ponchos, shawls, and cardigans (see Chapter 4 for newer arm covers). Just realize that anything that adds another layer has the potential to be fattening.

You probably don't want to hear this, but your best course of action is to keep buff the old-fashioned way: taking the time to work out (Michelle Obama does, at least four times a week), so you can flaunt sculpted shoulders all year long. How does Michelle do it? Read on.

> You probably don't want to hear this, but your best course of action is to keep buff the old-fashioned way: taking the time to work out (Michelle Obama does, at least four times a week), so you can flaunt sculpted shoulders all year long.

Every woman wants Michelle Obama's buff shoulders and arms. Sure, they're defined and chiseled but not to the extreme. *Women's Health* magazine reports that Michelle works out about four times a week with a trainer, and gets up at 5:30 a.m. to do it. Her workout includes one minute of hammercurls with dumbbells in alternating motions. And tricep pushdowns, 15–20 repetitions with 10–15-pound weights. Sounds doable. ●

SWAP-OUTS:
CHANGES TO MAKE RIGHT NOW

Instead of →	Choose
Boat necks	Scoop necks
Choker necklaces	Long chains
Crew-neck sweaters	Fine-gauge V-necks
Jackets with mandarin collars	Jackets with shawl collars
Mufflers, wrapped high	Long scarf draped loosely
Wide and dangly earrings	Stud earrings

HOW I TOOK OFF
TEN POUNDS
WITH THE FASHION FIT FORMULA

I recently had Janet Wood and Kathy McFadden visit my closet to demonstrate the brilliance of their Fashion Fit Formula, a business based on the fact that one size does not fit all. They figure out your most flattering lengths for skirts, pants, sleeves, jackets, tops, and necklaces; all in all, a dozen measurements, to the eighth of an inch, that they call "pivotal points." If you get your clothes tailored to their specifications, you will look ten (or more) pounds thinner. Worked for me.

They believe that whatever clothes you own can be customized to hit those exact places where your body will look its slimmest. Sign up for their program, and they will tell you how to measure yourself. Then send them the measurements and they'll do the calculations for your twelve pivotal points. When you have your specific lengths, share these with your tailor, and you will forever take the guesswork out of alterations. No matter how much weight you gain or lose, these pivotal points remain the same because they're based on your bone structure, which doesn't change no matter how much weight you gain. Love that. For your customized pivotal points, see their Web site, fashionfitformula.com.

10 THINGS THAT MAKE YOU LOOK FAT WITH A
Thick Neck + Broad Shoulders

1. Elizabethan ruffles and high collars of any kind. Unless you're Cate Blanchett playing Queen Elizabeth I or in the priesthood, avoid them!

2. An über-short cropped haircut or hair pulled back. This look only works if you are an Olympic swimmer with a killer body. Avoid very long flat hair, too, as it can have the reverse effect, aka the squat mushroom look.

3. Schlumping around, head down makes you look frumpy and hides your neck altogether. Walk around instead with your head up and shoulder blades so far back they're almost kissing.

4. Silk scarves wrapped and knotted around the neck, like Camp Fire Girls. If it's Hermès, wear the scarf as a belt or tie it on your bag . . . so much chicer.

5. Epaulettes. On military-inspired jackets, they're designed to make the upper body look more commanding—exactly what you don't need. Skip safari jackets for the same reason.

6. Boatneck tops with horizontal stripes. Both fattening on their own, together this double whammy cuts you off at the blades and packs on pounds.

7. The sweater-over-the-shoulder look. It once made you Ivy League cool. Now all it does is squish down your neck with another layer of heavy fabric.

8. Pashminas and shawls. Like ketchup on fries, these last-minute add-ons are very fattening, bringing bulk to where you need it least. Substitute long, loose scarves for the fashion look, cardigans to ward off the chill.

9. Backpacks and bulky shoulder bags. If you're hiking, okay, but for daily explorations in the urban jungle, you're unnecessarily packing pounds onto your frame. Haul daily essentials in a handheld tote instead.

10. Texting or sending e-mails on your iPhone or BlackBerry. Your head is down, tripling your chins and squashing your neck into your chest. Not a pretty sight.

JUST SAY NO
TO CHOKERS

When you are wearing a choker or any short necklace, you are in effect taking a yellow highlighter and drawing a circle around the circumference of your neck. Who needs that?

IF THE THOUGHT OF WEARING A CHOKER MAKES YOU GAG, NO NEED TO REQUEST THE HEIMLICH MANEUVER. Just a few minutes removing all chokers from your jewelry drawer will do it. A choker necklace is your jewelry nightmare because anything that disrupts the space between chin and collarbone will make your neck look stumpy. When you are wearing a choker or any short necklace, you are in effect taking a yellow highlighter and drawing a circle around the circumference of your neck. Who needs that?

And if your jewelry collection contains any type of collar necklace with matching earrings, break up the set and give away the collar. Worn together, those sets are so frumpy, and therefore lethal to your Fit Not Fat look.

The look in jewelry right now is piling on strands of chain, pearls, long beads, or diamonds by the yard! If they're a tangled mess, so much the better. Or, you can simplify and go solo with a single long standout pendant. The V-shape created by these necklaces will redirect the eye lower and read visually as a low neckline even if you wear a crewneck sweater. Skip the long earrings with this look.

Speaking of earrings, do yourself a favor and fall out of love with long earrings—dangly chandeliers, linear shoulder dusters, or oversized hoops—as they visually shorten that gap of space you're trying to create between earlobe and shoulder. Shorten your dangly earrings to no more than an inch.

WHAT SHOULD REMAIN IN YOUR STASH: medium-large hoop earrings, small teardrops, studs, and necklaces that hit mid-chest or longer. If you don't have them in your personal repertoire already, pendants, bibs, lariats, long chains of pearls, or dangling strands of (real or faux) diamonds will beautifully draw the eye down, down, down to where you want it. Need an excuse to buy yourself jewelry? You got it. ●

A NECK-FRIENDLY GUIDE TO JEWELS

═══

Good things to keep in your jewelry box

A delicate collarbone chain
with charm, locket, or pendant that drops to a V

A collection of adjustable link necklaces
that can be lengthened to mid-chest

A lariat necklace
to loop where you want

A bib with multiple beads
or strands coming off a single necklace

A waterfall, graduated, or cascade single necklace
with strands of beads or semi-precious stones

Tie-neck pearls

Long strands of linked chains, ropes, or beads
of similar length and type worn together

A pendant necklace,
cord, or chain, with an amulet or big charm

Stud earrings
small to large post in real or faux diamonds or pearls

Medium-large hoop earrings
not too tiny, not oversized

Teardrops earrings
with a small wire drop

HIGH FAT *vs.* NO FAT

→ Everyone sees your neck and shoulders . . . Elongate your neckline visually so that it appears more Penelope Cruz, less Incredible Hulk! Fight the urge to hide it behind a thick super-fattening turtleneck sweater (you're not fooling anyone). Instead, reveal it in a slenderizing deep-V.

HIGH FAT:
Ban the turtleneck and shoulder pads from your wardrobe. Pulling your hair back—or wearing a super short cut—only accentuates the problem.

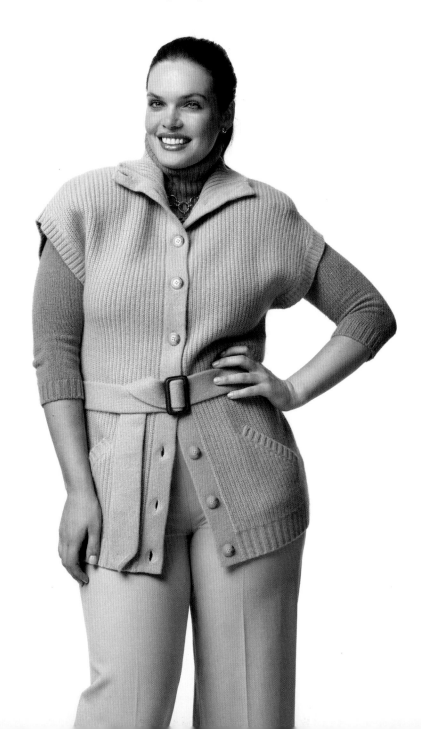

HOW FAST CAN YOU GIVE THESE AWAY?

HIGH FAT

× Chunky cabled sweaters

× Collarless boxy jackets

× Epaulettes

× Short puff-sleeve blouses

× Shoulder pads

× Turtlenecks

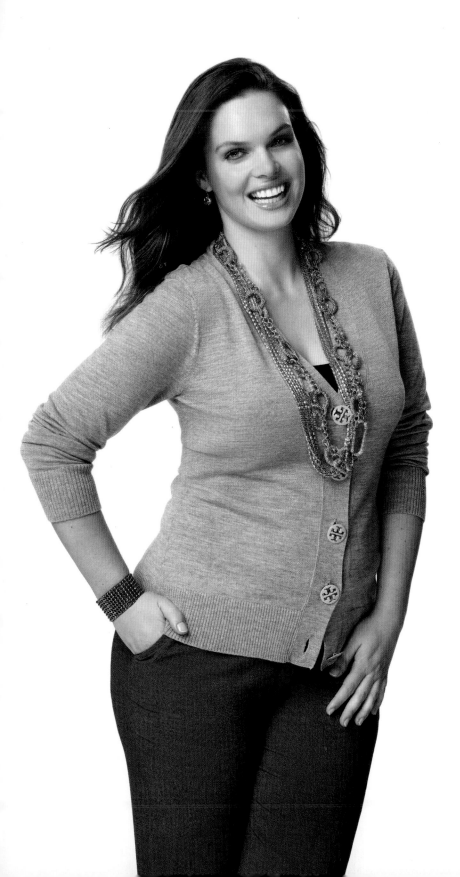

What a difference!

*From football hero to
slim and sexy shoulders;
from no neck to
vampire-bait.*

NO FAT:
Open up the area with
deep-V necklines. A
chic tangle of necklaces
draws the eye to the
smallest part of your torso.

YOU CAN'T HAVE
TOO MANY OF THESE!

NO FAT

√ Deep square-neck top or tank

√ Deep V-neck sweater

√ Hand-carried tote bags
and satchels

√ One-shoulder asymmetrical
dress

√ Scoop-neck dress with jeweled
neckline (no necklace needed!)

√ Wrap dress with V neckline

Thinner by Tonight!

INSTANT GRATIFICATION

Snip out those shoulder pads!
You don't need them—not even little bitty ones. Do this to every jacket and sweater you own—and if there is excess fabric, have the tailor make the alteration. Pads are for women who don't have enough shoulders. Best to recycle them as shoe shapers.

Create a crisp new frame.
Throw a black, tailored, fitted jacket, open, over a white, bright, or light-colored V-neck tee. The dark, angular cut of the jacket reduces body weight at the shoulders, while the contrasting V-neck creates the illusion of a longer neck.

Break up your twinsets.
They can really look frumpy, so substitute a sexy camisole or tank for that matching crew or turtleneck shell.

Unbutton everything!
Button-front shirts, blouses, and shirtdresses to above your bra, and pull the neckline open to form a V. Raise the collar up in the back to help keep the neck open.

Pin a pretty jeweled brooch at bra level
to anchor partially unbuttoned shirts and cardigans to a V. The weight of the brooch will help keep the neckline open.

Loosen up. Take yoga, Pilates, or stretch class.
Or pick up a DVD on yoga, Pilates, or stretching next time you're in Costco. Your body will be more aware of what it feels like to stand upright. Your posture will be improved. You'll look like you've grown an inch or two.

Tilt your head slightly in conversation, but especially when taking pictures.
Press the top of your tongue to the roof of your mouth, too, as you smile to pull up chin dangle. The greatest portrait photographers in the world tell their subjects that before clicking.

THICK NECK SOLUTIONS

IF YOU'RE PETITE…

• SEEK OUT DRESSES AND TOPS WITH EMBELLISHED V-NECK OR SCOOP NECK-LINES. That way you don't have to add yet another piece.

• CHOOSE STRETCH FABRICS with a little Lycra® or spandex to ensure better fit when dealing with lower necklines.

• GO FOR SUPPLE COWLS, DRAPED NECKLINES, AND V-NECK SLEEVELESS TOPS AND DRESSES. Get rid of scrunch-down turtles and boxy crews that overwhelm smaller proportions and make you look shorter and wider.

• BEWARE OF ORIGAMI FOLDS. A long torso is required to pull these off.

• WATCH THE KEYHOLE NECK. Keyhole necklines are an open slit, circle, or oval shape on the neckline, usually topped with a button or hook closure. Often the size of the keyhole is too deep on a petite and reveals too much.

IF YOU'RE SIZE 14 & UP…

• BUY SWEATERS IN BLACK, GRAY, NAVY, OR CHOCOLATE. You'll look ten pounds heavier in a sweater that is light or bright.

• PLAY WITH DRAMATIC NECKLINES—you can handle it. Portrait collar jackets with a rich retro look, deep square necklines, crisp white notch-collar shirts, and wide-strap beaded neck scoops are wait-ing for you.

• FEM UP WITH BLOUSES THAT TIE LOW ON THE CHEST IN A LARGE, LOOSE BOW; they can give you a fash-ion edge.

• BRING SEXY BACK. Structured fitted dresses with scoop necks or shape-hugging tops with stretch will beautifully accentuate your curves.

• STUDY PHOTOS OF QUEEN LATIFAH. More often than not, the Queen nails it.

WHAT ELSE YOU CAN DO TO
SAVE YOUR NECK

We have to continue to thank witty Nora Ephron for creating buzz around this previously ignored body part with her delicious collection of essays, *I Feel Bad About My Neck*. Compared to breasts and butts, the neck never got its share of press, until Nora wrote so amusingly about aging. While this chapter is not about old necks but fat necks, a neck with folds of excess skin due to aging is fattening. So you want to preventatively take care of your neck to delay the aging process, and if it's too late—i.e., you indeed have rolls of neck—there are extreme measures that can be taken at the dermatologist's and plastic surgeon's office.

ERADICATE NECK NEGLECT.
We lavish attention on faces and bodies, but necks get no respect. This is probably because we leave them out when we're cleansing and moisturizing our faces every morn-ing and evening, and when we're in the shower or bath, we don't want to spend a lot of time around the neck because it will ruin our blown-dry hair under the shower cap.

Should the neck be treated as part of our face? Or body? Start by treating your neck as an extension of your face, says San Francisco dermatologist Dr. Seth Matarasso, who suggests "cleansing, moisturizing, and wearing a broad-spectrum UVA/UVB sunscreen daily on the front and back of your neck from chest up to hairline." (Don't feel bad about not doing the back of the neck. Who knew?) "Before bed, Retin-A (by prescription) will eliminate sun damage on the neck, especially around the sides, where most women scrimp on sunscreen."

TAKE YOUR CALCIUM.
The neck is the most flexible, supple part of the spine, but as we age, extreme bone loss in the form of osteoporosis can result in a shorter, hunched neck and shoulder silhou-ette. This can begin as early as your late fifties!

Estrogen deficiency is the usual cause of bone loss, and women can lose as much as 20 percent of their bone mass in the five years follow-ing menopause. A bone density test plus a medical evaluation to determine the degree of bone loss can determine your best course of action, but a high intake of calcium plus vitamin D (which facilitates the absorption of calcium) and bump-ing up your weight-bearing exer-cise at least five times a week can help. Pump iron to keep your bones strong and healthy. No one wants osteopenia—or worse, the shrinking hunched-over camel-hump that sig-nals degeneration. ●

Going to Extremes: *Neck Work*

Do your face and neck look like they belong to two different people? The neck often ages faster than the face, says New York plastic surgeon Alan Matarasso, MD, FACS. "A lot of women who began using a sun-screen on their faces as early as a decade or two ago continued to tan their neck and bodies, and the con-trast between neck and face is incredible!" The skin on your neck is thin, fragile, and susceptible to UVA/UVB rays and, no, the overhanging ledge of your chin does not protect you. Your neck has had nearly as much sun exposure as your face and, in most cases, more—having gone defenseless for so long. Don't feel bad about your neck . . . at least you have options.

FOR SUBTLE NECK TIGHTENING. If your problem is slack, not fat, Manhattan dermatologist Gervaise

DO YOU REALLY NEED A NECK CREAM?

Dr. Seth Matarasso doesn't think so. Neither does a dear friend of mine, who is responsible for creating a hugely successful skin-care line, yet admits that neck creams are just a way to get you to buy another product.

But anyone in the beauty biz who has a special neck cream in his or her line will try to convince you that the skin on the neck is so much different than the skin on your face! Listen, if spending $80 or more is the only thing that will compel you to care for your neck, go for it. Most of us don't want another beauty product out on the counter when something that we already own will do the same trick.

Neck products essentially use the same ingredients as facial treatments. Using your face cream on your neck, too, is fine when neck and face have the same skin quality. Sometimes neck treatments are more occlusive than face treatments because you don't wear makeup over them. You might want to consider a different product for face and neck when the skin on your neck and face don't match. Say your neck skin is very dehydrated, lined, or crepey and your facial skin is not. In that case, a thicker cream with a higher concentration of barrier ingredients might be good to slather on your neck. High up on the label should be ingredients that prevent moisture loss, such as mineral oil, silicones, petrolatum, shea butter, or natural oils like almond or jojoba.

Gerstner, MD, says that she has seen wonderful results with the new and improved Fraxel laser for neck and chest. Numbing cream is required to ease the pain of a hot light passing over your skin as it resurfaces it (in other words, as it burns off a few layers). "It addresses slack neck texture, chicken skin, creped skin, and fine lines but does require five visits a month apart for results to show," she says. After Fraxel, you may not want to go out on the town that evening, as you may still be red and swollen. Unlike most injectibles, Fraxel's results are permanent. If you have a big event like a reunion or wedding, it will provide the appearance of a tighter neck and jaw without major surgery.

FOR A SCRAWNY SAGGY NECK AND DROOPY JAW. The Botox neck-lift is another treatment option if fat

BRILLIANT BUYS

COSTUME JEWELRY

Ann Taylor; Ann Taylor, anntaylor.com.

Chico's; Chico's, chicos.com.

J.Crew; J.Crew, jcrew.com.

Aqua; Bloomingdale's, bloomingdales.com.

Kenneth Jay Lane; Bloomingdale's; bloomingdales.com.

RJ Graziano; Bloomingdale's; hsn.com.

Sequin; Nordstrom, nordstrom.com.

FINE JEWELRY

Lisa Stein; lastein.com.

Ippolita; ippolita.com, neimanmarcus.com, saks.com.

NECK CREAMS

Shiseido White Lucent Brightening Serum for Neck and Décolletage, $75; Sephora, macys.com.

Vichy Laboratoires Neovadiol Gf Day, $48; CVS, vichyusa.com.

SPF FOR NECK

Aveeno SPF 30 Ultra-Calming Daily Moisturizer, $14.99; mass retailers, drugstore.com.

Olay Complete SPF 30 Defense Daily UV Moisturizer—Sensitive Skin, $14.99; mass retailers, drugstore.com.

Neutrogena Anti-Oxidant Age Reverse Day Lotion SPF 20, $19.99; mass retailers, drugstore.com.

---

is not an issue. Why? Botox will relax the platysma bands of muscle under the skin of your neck. It's good for that little dribble of fat under the chin and obvious cords. Botox injections from the chin to the clavicle will lift neck skin and fat pads as the platysma muscle is relaxed. This injectible muscle freezer has a cumulative effect; the more you do, the longer it lasts. It does take a few days for the full effect to kick in, and it's not permanent, so expect to go back every three or four months. "Easy and great," Dr. Gerstner calls it. "Just injections. No risk. Worst case—when you eat a giant piece of steak, it could be a little tight to swallow." Gulp.

TO REMOVE NECK FAT. Traditional tumescent lipo can remove excess fat. "Lipo is an option for youngish necks with fat and no sag," says Dr. Matarasso. "It requires a small incision under the chin, the fat is suctioned out, and you're done." You go home with your face in an elastic sling and you can expect swelling and bruising for about two weeks, with final results in a month.

FOR TIGHTENING, FAT REMOVAL, AND DROOP. A neck-lift, often done on women in their fifties and sixties who have saggy skin, fat, and loss of firmness and definition, addresses all three concerns as it tightens and not only removes fat but excess skin. The fat pad under the platysma muscle is removed, the platysma muscle tightened and (in some cases) shortened, while hanging skin is trimmed. Dr. Matarasso always does a neck-lift at the same time as a face-lift but, "If you have such great facial architecture that all you have is a saggy neck, we now do a neck-lift or platysmaplasty on its own to refresh things," he says, describing it as "a three-level operation. We make an incision, vacuum out the fat between the skin and the muscle, tighten the muscle or maybe even remove a little of it, and trim the excess skin before suturing up behind the ears." The reason that lipo on its own isn't enough on an older neck is because when fat is sucked out, the underlying muscle bands, hanging glands, and loose skin can show up even worse after the fatty cushion is removed with lipo. ●

Vows *for* Thick Neck + Broad Shoulders

- ☐ **I WILL** make the V-neck my neckline of choice.

- ☐ **I WILL** give away all my turtlenecks.

- ☐ **I WILL** donate my big, dangly chandelier earrings.

- ☐ **I WILL** show some love to my neck and treat it as well as I treat my face.

- ☐ **I WILL** show off my shoulders in asymmetrical dresses and tops.

- ☐ **I WILL** get up and take a walk after sitting at the computer for hours to counteract the effects of forward schlumping.

- ☐ **I WILL** stand up straight and try to walk with shoulders back, summoning up my inner supermodel.

DON'T YOU DARE...

Wear a high-neck puffer coat in the winter.
Your neck will disappear. Remember the Michelin Man!

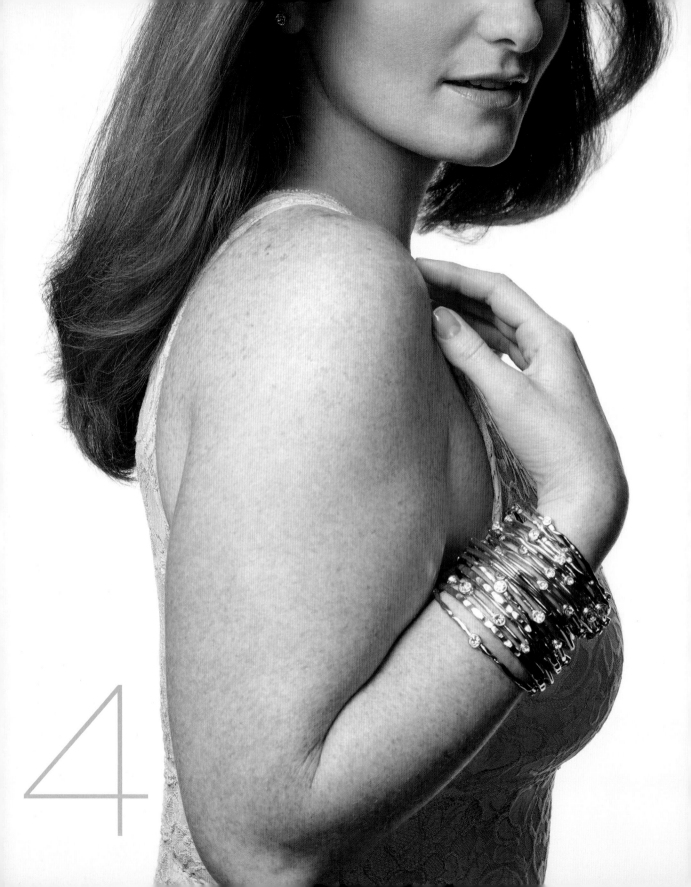

Arm Flap

AKA
batwings,
arm dangle,
flab flaps,
porkchop arms,
lambchops,
grandma flab,
bingo wings,
mozzarella
arms, arm
waggle, big
guns, flabbies,
teacher arms

YOU KNOW YOU HAVE IT WHEN...
You refuse to play tennis or volleyball... You wear a jacket or sweater in 90-degree heat... You do the Queen Elizabeth royal wave from elbow to wrist... When you raise your arm to signal a taxi, you hope you don't see anyone you know... You look like you're wearing a dolman sweater when nude...

→ How many times have you passed up a totally cute dress on the rack because you need, want, have to have sleeves? I wish more designers would realize that most women, especially those of us over forty, are either always cold or not happy with our upper arms.

Maybe designers *do* realize this; they just want us to buy that second piece for arm cover. On a recent shopping trip, I fell in love with a sleeveless purple print silk shift. The dress was not outrageously priced, but the wet-look patent leather cropped motorcycle jacket that I needed for arm cover was more than double the price of the dress! Granted, the addition of the jacket gave the outfit an edgier look, but would I have preferred to buy just one piece that day and save myself a hefty credit card charge? What do you think? So not only is arm dangle a shopping challenge, it's expensive. Think of all the wraps, shawls, scarves, shrugs, cardis, boleros, pashminas, capelets, capes, ponchos, blouses, jackets, and coats you've invested in over the years—just because of that jiggle! Which is all the more reason to make those bat wings fly away.

Unlike other body issues covered in this book, arm flap doesn't necessarily mean that you're overweight. In fact, arm flap can happen to any grown woman who thinks that she can get away with not working her triceps (that used to be me). Or,

lished tank tops year-round. Arm role models like Kelly Ripa without a ripple or drip of flesh go sleeveless as much as possible, even in winter. This right to not only bare arms but to flaunt them has become a status symbol of the fit, but instead of being frustrated at having to look at Kelly's arms in the middle of a February blizzard, we can choose to be inspired.

(see Going to Extremes, page 64).

If you are a lawyer, a banker, or an executive in a conservative business, you'll want to cover your arms in the office, as it's more professional. You rarely see a news anchor, such as Katie Couric, Diane Sawyer, Meredith Vieira, or Leslie Stahl, go sleeveless on-air. The same dress code goes for power politicos such

Unlike other body issues covered in this book, arm flap doesn't necessarily mean that you're overweight. In fact, arm flap can happen to any grown woman who thinks that she can get away with not working her triceps (that used to be me).

it can happen to those who have shed an excessive amount of weight and is quite common after gastric bypass surgery. It's what happens when loose skin—without the fat to cling to anymore—is just left flapping in the wind. You don't have to be fat to be flabby (or flappy, for that matter). Think of flapping arms, and you picture an older woman—a schoolteacher from the 1950s writing on a chalkboard or an old-fashioned granny in a housedress.

Today, more women are weight lifting, and workplace dress codes are more casual than ever, so everyone who can makes it a point to flaunt her tight, toned arms in body-skimming T-shirts, sleeveless shifts and sweaters, or cute little embel-

I know that you didn't pick up this book to learn about exercise, and that you already know this, but I do have to say that the best (and cheapest) way to rid yourself of arm flap is working your triceps (see What Else You Can Do About the Flappies, page 58). And the good news is that arms are relatively easy to tone up, as they really respond to a little attention. Weight-bearing exercises, such as picking up a dumbbell, are so much better for your muscle mass, your metabolism, your strength, and your posture than any surgical alternative. An arm lift, for example, leaves a seam of scarring down the inner arm, so you're back to where you started, still needing arm cover to hide the seam

as Hillary Clinton. They have an endless supply of jackets and coats that convey authority, conveniently taking the issue of arm dangle off the table. Still, some jackets—make that sleeves—are better than others at hiding the evidence.

But first, you have to ask yourself, should you—or shouldn't you—go sleeveless? ●

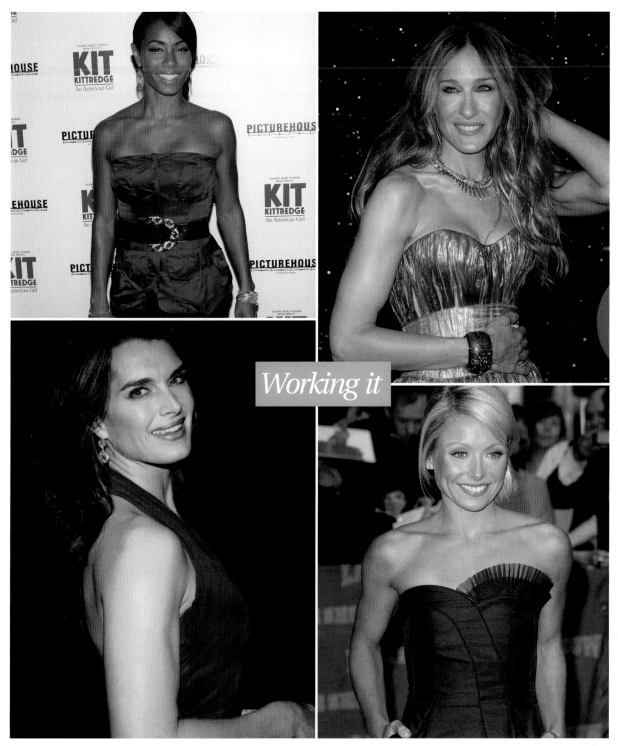

Working it

Women who aren't afraid to pick up a dumbbell.
Clockwise from top left: JADA PINKETT SMITH, SARAH JESSICA PARKER, KELLY RIPA, AND BROOKE SHIELDS

This chapter is about arm flap, but most of the advice will also apply to heavy arms, if that better describes your upper arm issue. Either way, think about how you feel about going sleeveless in public. Carrie Fisher says in her one-woman show *Wishful Drinking,* "I haven't been naked in thirteen years, sleeveless in twenty." Maybe this is a moot point and you cover your arms anyway because you're always cold, even in summer in overly air-conditioned buildings, stores, restaurants, and movie theaters. Maybe your comfort level is occasion driven. How self-conscious are you? After all, you know best how much flapping you have going on!

If you're confident enough to say that a little arm bounce-back is no big deal, good for you, skip this chapter. I'm certainly not okay about flaunting my flap when I know that people are really looking at me. When I'm on TV or giving a speech, I want to be covered. But there are exceptions. When I spoke at the Biltmore Fashion Park in Phoenix, Arizona, and the temperature hit 100 degrees, off went the jacket! I revealed my arms for all to see in a print silk top because wearing a leather jacket over it in that heat would only call attention to the situation—as in, *Is she nuts? What is she trying to hide?* Now, if I'm just running around the neighborhood doing errands and it's broiling hot out, I will go sleeveless rather than sweat it out over a little flab.

Please don't feel that you absolutely must always keep your arms covered. Maybe the only one who notices your arm flab is you. But, on the other hand, who's more important than you? If you feel more comfortable covered, you need a strategy.

YOUR DRESS-THINNER STRATEGY
for Arm Flap

→WHETHER THE ARM IN QUESTION IS as mushy as a ball of fresh mozzarella or bigger and more muscular than you'd like, you want to wear fabrics that don't amplify the upper arm but instead those that gently skim the skin and go with the flow—soft matte jerseys, rayons, crepes, and washed silks.

At the same time, you want to divert attention downward, to the part of your arm that is firmer, smaller, bonier—from your elbow to your wrist.

FIRST, LOOK THROUGH THE LIST OF HIGH-FAT ARM COVERS (see page 62) and weed out all the offenders hanging in your closet. While you're at it, toss every sleeve that makes you feel like it's cutting off your circulation. You don't need that kind of pressure!

PAY ATTENTION TO SLEEVE SHAPE AND SLEEVE LENGTH like you never have before. With laser-like focus, hunt down the universally flattering three-quarter-

length sleeve (which hits midway between elbow and wrist). Also flattering is a bracelet sleeve (slightly longer than the three-quarter, it stops right above the wrist), and an elbow-length diagonal sleeve where the high part of the sleeve hits the outer arm. Ask your tailor to customize your sleeves so that they angle at your exact slimming proportions and see what a big difference this little adjustment can make.

THE FUN PART
Play magician, with a bag of tricks to divert all eyes to your wrist and hands. Now you have a new excuse to bejewel yourself with glamorous wrist candy. Knock yourself out shopping for fabulous bangles, bracelets, cuffs, statement watches, and cocktail rings. And don't stop there. If you have beautiful hands, draw attention to them with manicured nails and dramatic dark polish. This strategy for drawing attention away from the upper arms works for every woman with arm flap—size 2 or 22. And now, a crash course on sleeves. ●

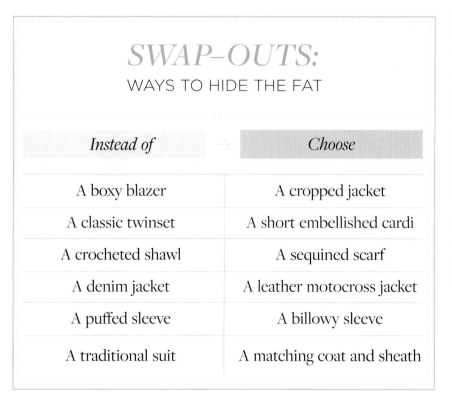

SWAP-OUTS:
WAYS TO HIDE THE FAT

Instead of →	*Choose*
A boxy blazer	A cropped jacket
A classic twinset	A short embellished cardi
A crocheted shawl	A sequined scarf
A denim jacket	A leather motocross jacket
A puffed sleeve	A billowy sleeve
A traditional suit	A matching coat and sheath

AN ARM-FRIENDLY GUIDE TO SLEEVES

Your most dependable arm-slimmer will always be the three-quarter sleeve, but high-drama fuller sleeves are now the height of fashion. If you're tall, don't miss out on these airy, fuller sleeves. If you're petite, you probably know that the fuller sleeves might overwhelm you. But whatever your size, the trick is to make sure the billowy sleeve is attached to a slim-fitting jacket, top, blouse, sweater, dress, or coat, as you don't want to be billowing all over. On the right piece, these new full sleeves can be better camouflage than a humongous sweatshirt or oversized sweater, which will just make you look shapeless all over and wider than you really are. As you are well aware, fuller arms need sleeves that fit comfortably. The higher-set the sleeve, the tighter it will be. The iconic Chanel tweed jacket, known for its snug sleeves, is often a deal breaker for those with muscular or otherwise bulky upper arms—as in, "Oh, forget it. I can't even get my arms in there!" Petites, on the other hand, love the close fit.

Balloon
Big, billowy sleeve

Bell
Fitted sleeve that flares
toward elbow or wrist

Bishop
Long sleeve fitted on top,
fuller at bottom, ending
in a cuff

Bracelet-length
Cropped two or three
inches above wrist

Dolman or batwing
Very deep, wide armhole
narrows at wrist

Elbow-length
An elongated half sleeve
to the elbow

Flutter
Ruffled or wavy-edged
loose short sleeve

Kimono
Deep armhole, square,
structured sleeve

Lantern
Fitted to mid—upper arm then
widens in a lampshade shape

Poet
Fitted sleeve that
dramatically flares or
ruffles at forearm

Raglan
Seam extends toward neck
in a curve for moveability

**Tailored pinstriped
long-sleeve**
In French or contrast
cuffs, a crisp shirt with
attention-getting
wrist treatment

Three-quarter
Below the elbow at
mid-forearm

WHAT ELSE YOU CAN DO
ABOUT THE FLAPPIES

After forty, every woman needs to do a few simple, easy exercises to work her triceps.
It's not only about buff, enviable arms, but about arm strength.

Why does the skin underneath our arms get so loosey-goosey? I asked Dr. Pamela Peeke, MD, author of *New York Times* bestsellers *Fight Fat After Forty, Body for Life for Women,* and *Fit to Live.* Dr. Peeke has been called a nutri-shrink, because she's a medical doc who deals with both the mind and the body as she looks at the mental and physical fitness of the whole woman. "A lot of the reason these flappies happen has to do with disuse because lifting overhead is something that most women don't do on a regular basis," she says. We lift bags of groceries, we lift babies up to a point. But when does a woman push over her head, unless we're in an airplane or reaching on a store shelf?" Another reason is hormonal. "It's a postmenopausal elasticity issue associated with estrogen withdrawal. You can take some of the punch out of it with hormones, but hormones are not going to do it on their own."

After forty, every woman needs to do a few simple, easy exercises to work her triceps. Do your arms get tired blow-drying your hair or reading the newspaper? Amp up your arm strength. "If you stay on top of it, the amount of skin hang will be minimized," Dr. Peeke promises. Here are her no-brainers (you'll find more exercises—such as my favorite tricep kickbacks—in her *Body for Life for Women*).

"LEARN TO DO A SIMPLE BENT-KNEE PUSH-UP. You're going to be hitting triceps, biceps, chest, shoulder, abdomen, and butt—six muscles. You can do it anywhere. Start with one or two—in good form."

"DO A DIP. Grab a stable chair — not one with wheels. Put your palms on each side of the chair, take your behind off the chair, bend the knees, put feet flat on the ground and hoist your behind up and down."

"THERE'S ONE I CALL BRUSHING YOUR HAIR. Use one of those three-ounce tubes that look like jump ropes. With one foot on the rope, bring the arm straight above the head in front of the body."

AND IF THOSE DON'T DO IT FOR YOU, HOW ABOUT JUMPING ROPE, PUNCHING OUT A PUNCHING BAG, OR SWIMMING THE BUTTERFLY STROKE? It doesn't matter what you do, just as long as you do something consistently. Health-wise, you'll increase your muscle mass so that you'll burn more calories every day and help speed up your metabolism. You don't need to look as sinewy as Madonna; just tone your arms enough so you can see what lies beneath. Every woman looks better with a little muscle definition. Just do it. ●

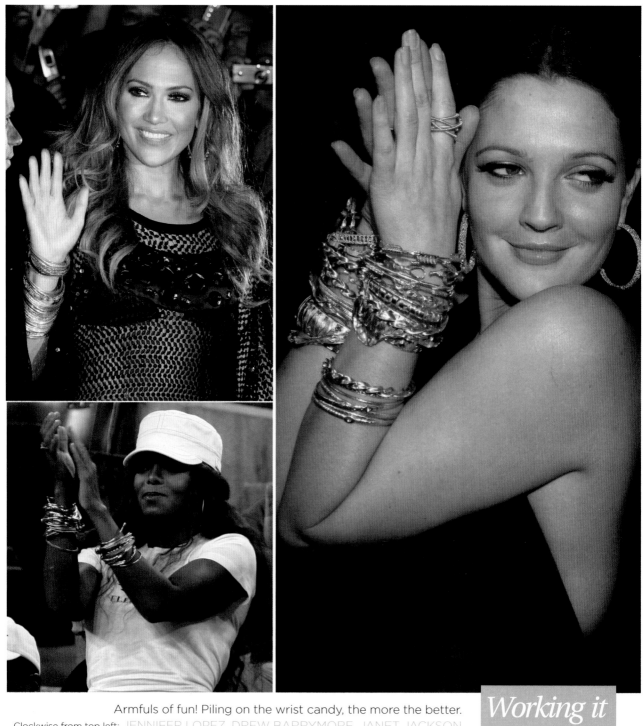

Armfuls of fun! Piling on the wrist candy, the more the better.
Clockwise from top left: JENNIFER LOPEZ, DREW BARRYMORE, JANET JACKSON

Working it

10 THINGS THAT MAKE YOU LOOK FAT WITH *Arm Flap*

1. Second skin fabrics that reveal all

2. Shiny, thick, stiff fabrics that magnify arms

3. Layering more than one sleeve on top of another

4. Compressing the flesh by crossing arms on top of each other

5. Holding your hands straight down at your sides

6. A banded sleeve that draws a virtual line across your arm

7. Short sleeves with pockets, tab closures, zippers, logos and other attention-getting doodads

8. A puffer coat with a horizontal seam across the upper arm

9. An upper-arm bracelet or tattoo

10. A furry arm—bleach it, wax it, or laser off the fuzz

HIGH FAT *vs.* NO FAT

→ You don't have to be fat to have arm flap. It happens to skinny minnies, too. If reverberations of loose flab doesn't motivate you to make regular dates with a dumbbell, you will wake one day and find yourself gravitating toward clothes with sleeves—the longer, more billowy, the better.

HIGH FAT:
A peasant is not so pleasant when its banded puff sleeve hits you across the widest part of your arm, especially in a contrasting color.

HOW FAST CAN YOU GIVE THESE AWAY?

HIGH FAT

- × Cap or puff sleeves
- × Knit suit jackets
- × Sequin muscle tees
- × Shrunken "baby" tees
- × Sleeveless or strapless dresses
- × Tube tops

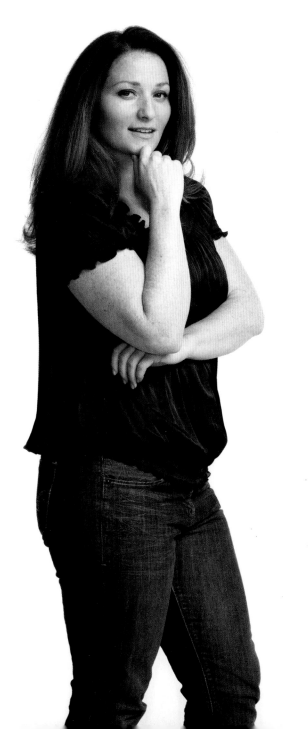

NO FAT:
If you're tall, balance long, loose sleeves with a torso-hugging style that shows off your shape. Petites: You do better in a slim-fitting jacket or cardigan.

YOU CAN'T HAVE TOO MANY OF THESE!

NO FAT

√ Billowy jersey full sleeves

√ Shrugs and capes

√ Slouchy sweaters and tees with V or scoop necks

√ Tailored dress/cardigan combos

√ Three-quarter sleeves

√ Tunics with straight, roomy sleeves

Thinner by Tonight!

INSTANT GRATIFICATION

Hands on hips, Batgirl-style or at least one hand on a hip, elongates the arms and makes the most of your muscle definition. Models and actresses know that this creates maximal space between your arm and torso.

Compress the jiggle in a Tres Sleek De Quart Sleeve (see Brilliant Buys, page 68).

Slightly faux-tan your arms. The glow will appear to reduce your arm size, wipe out little white bumps on elbows, and even out age spots. Do face and legs, too, so you're fully blended.

Slip on an off-the-shoulder top that plays up your shoulders and neck while covering up upper arms.

Throw on a long scarf, a mass of necklaces, a brooch, a zipper sweater, or a ruffled blouse . . . Front and center details draw the eye front and center, away from your outer silhouette.

Fake three-quarter sleeves with a band that holds sleeves in place (see Brilliant Buys, page 68).

Pile on the wrist candy: cuffs, thick bangles, stacks of silver and gold bracelets, a big watch.

Slip on gloves: driving gloves in warmer weather, cold weather gloves in winter.

Work your triceps minutes before you leave the house. This really does work. Try it.

Going to Extremes: *Arm Work*

If you're beginning to think that a family of bats somehow is hidden in your genealogical past, you do have other options. For serious skin hang, as a result of a fifty-plus-pound weight loss, there is lipo and plastic surgery. These are not substitutes for exercise, and every surgery (even lipo) is risky. No one wants her obit to read: cause of death—surgery for arm flab. But here is what dermatologists and plastic surgeons offer.

AT THE DERM'S OFFICE. Dr. Deborah Sarnoff, whose practice is in Greenvale, New York, says LaserLipo is excellent for flappy arms because "there is no cutting, no ugly scars. The loose skin contracts and tightens; it's not just a matter of melting fat. If all you did was melt fat, the air would be let out of the balloon so to speak, and the skin would still hang, actually even more than before." Downtime: Normal activity can be resumed in a couple days; strenuous activity, about a month. You need to wear a compression garment (think sports bra with

ARM FLAP SOLUTIONS

IF YOU'RE PETITE...

- STICK TO A SLIM-STRUC-TURED SLEEVE on a jacket, shirt, or shirtdress.

- SIMPLE SCULPTED TOPS AND DRESSES in soft, pretty solids will make you look thinner.

- SAY NO TO SLEEVES WITH FRILLS, EPAULETTES, BIG BOWS,

HAMBURGER-PATTY-SIZED BUTTONS—they're just fattening sauces that pack on pounds.

- STEER CLEAR OF EXTREME DOLMAN AND KIMONO SLEEVES or you'll look like you're about to take flight. Look for mod-ified versions on tops and dresses that really nip in at the waist.

- WHEN YOU FIND BASICS IN THE RIGHT PROPORTIONS, STOCK UP. A three-quarter sleeve on someone five-foot-seven will likely be a long sleeve on you.

- ASK YOURSELF, "AM I WEAR-ING THIS? OR IS THIS WEARING ME?" It's easy to drown in too much fabric, pattern, accessories.

IF YOU'RE SIZE 14 & UP...

- START A TUNIC COLLECTION. The easy-fitting sleeve looks Fit Not Fat over slim pants, capris, or jeans. Check out Tory Burch, Tibi, Chico's, or Talbots.

- EXPERIMENT WITH SLEEVES: dolman, bishop, raglan, bell, kimono, flutter.

- THROW ON A CAPE, especially if you're on the tall side.

- LOOK THINNER AND LONGER BY KEEPING TOPS AND BOT-TOMS IN THE SAME COLOR TONE. High contrast between your upper and lower body is high fat.

---

three-quarter-length sleeves) to reduce swelling.

If your issue is just fat and not hanging drapey skin, standard arm lipo in which excess fat is suctioned out may be enough. Joan Rivers, who writes about having this done in her book *Men Are Stupid . . . And They Like Big Boobs*, recommends it for younger women who still have elasticity. Downtime: You'll wear the compression garment from one to two weeks.

Yet to be FDA-approved (at press time), says Dr. Sarnoff, is Bodytite by Invasix, a form of radio-frequency-

assisted lipo, which also melts fat and tightens skin via heat. One probe is inserted under the skin to melt fat and a second probe is placed on the surface of the skin for tightening.

AT THE PLASTIC SURGEON'S. An arm-lift, which is called a brachioplasty, may be necessary after massive weight loss and is a common follow-up to gastric bypass surgery as it can remove an extreme amount of excess skin, says → *continued on page 68*

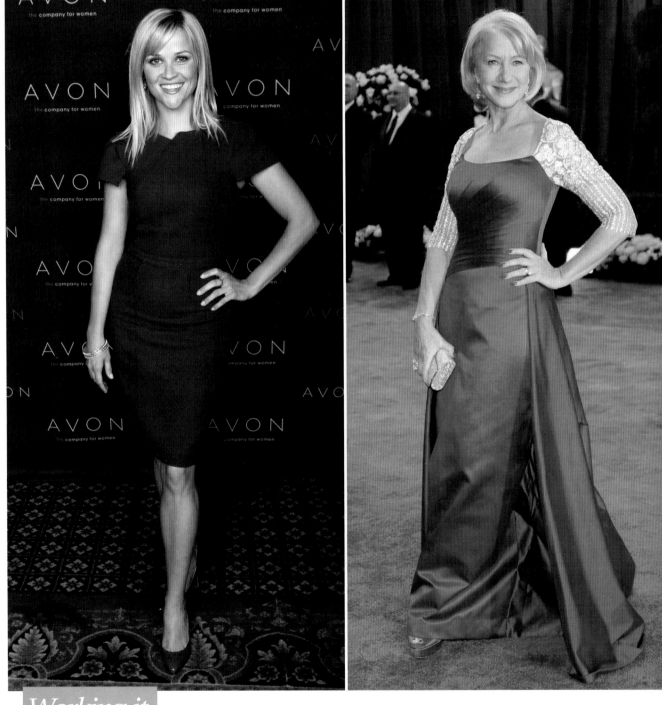

Working it

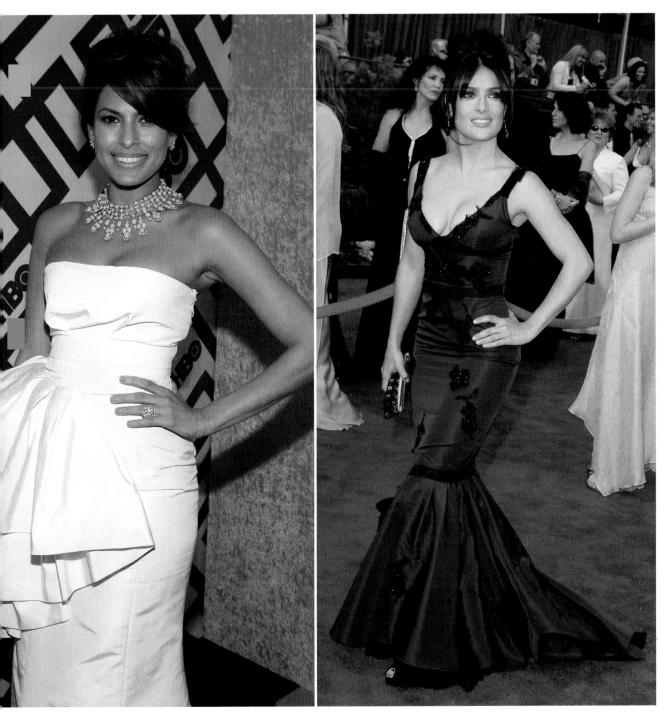

Strike a pose. The hand on hip trick is an award-winning move. And every star knows it.
REESE WITHERSPOON, HELEN MIRREN, EVA MENDES, SALMA HAYEK

BRILLIANT BUYS

ANTI-AGING BODY CLEANSER

Olay Total Effects 7-in-1 Advanced Anti-Aging Body Wash, $5.99; mass retailers, drugstore.com.

FIRMING MOISTURIZER

Aveeno Positively Ageless Firming Body Lotion, $8.99; mass retailers, drugstore.com.

INSTANT SLEEVES

Fashion Fit Formula Arm Bands, $10; fashionfitformula.com. Stretchy bands in silver, black, or gold hide in the folds of your sleeves and keep them in place.

SHAPEWEAR FOR ARMS

Spanx On Top and In Control Draped V Long Sleeve, $98; spanx.com.

Slimpressions The Haves or The Have-Nots, sleevage control top with or without cleavage compression, $72; slimpressions.com.

Tres Sleek De Quart Arm Shaper Sleeve elbow length, $21; tressleek.com. A form-fitting set of black stretchy sleeves that controls arm flap.

ARM TONING EXERCISERS

SPRI Xertube® Resistance Band, Door Attachment, and Exercise Chart, $9.99; amazon.com.

HAND LOTION

Bliss High Intensity Hand Cream To Go, $8; Sephora, sephora.com.

Burt's Bees Aloe and Witch Hazel Hand Sanitizer, $4.99; mass retailers, drugstore.com.

MANICURES

Essie Nail Polish Spaghetti Strap, Miss Matched, High Maintenance, Starter Wife, Room with a View, My Way, $8 each; Ulta, drugstore.com.

OPI Nail Lacquers It's a Girl, Isn't That Precious, $8.50 each; Ulta, opi.com.

New York plastic surgeon Dr. Alan Matarasso. While he's doing a brachioplasty, he adds liposuction to remove any remaining excess fat. And that little puffy piece of flab between your boobs and armpit, called an "arm scallop," can also be excised. Yes, this "enables women to wear skinny sleeve tops, jackets, and sweaters without a stuffed-sausage look," according to Dr. Matarasso, but not without a trace. "This surgery leaves big, grotesque scars from elbow to armpit, six to ten inches in length," he warns. For moderate excess skin, he can do a shorter incision in the armpit. Downtime: at least two weeks.

PS: I have a friend who lost more than a hundred pounds on gastric bypass and had this surgery (not from Dr. Matarasso). She describes the downtime and aftermath as "nasty . . . your arms are drained, and you have to constantly wrap them in gauzy material. It's been three years and I still have thick red scars from my elbow to armpit. I lost feeling in my arms and have nerve damage, so I'm still seeing an acupuncturist. Having someone touch my arms is painful. This wreaks havoc on your sex life." Dumbbells, anyone? ●

Vows *for* Arms

☐ **I WILL NOT** wear sleeves that are so tight that they hurt.

☐ **I WILL** only wear lightweight, sleeveless pieces under jackets and cardigans.

☐ **I WILL** buy three-quarter-length sweaters in multiples.

☐ **I WILL** donate all my short-sleeve polo shirts to charity.

☐ **I WILL** say that I'm "a little chilly" when asked to remove my coat/jacket/sweater rather than mention arm flap.

☐ **I WILL** put the old pashmina out to pasture.

☐ **I WILL** swap the denim jacket for a shrug.

☐ **I WILL** freshen up my summer look with a flattering tunic.

☐ **I WILL NEVER** wear a sleeveless dress with elbow-length gloves like they show on the runway.

☐ **I WILL** remove the tattoo from my upper arm.

DON'T YOU DARE...

Go sleeveless when wearing pants or jeans. When baring arms, it's always better to wear a skirt or dress. That way, everyone will be looking at your bare legs or thighs. It's the fastest way to switch the focus to your legs, which may be more shapely than your upper arms.

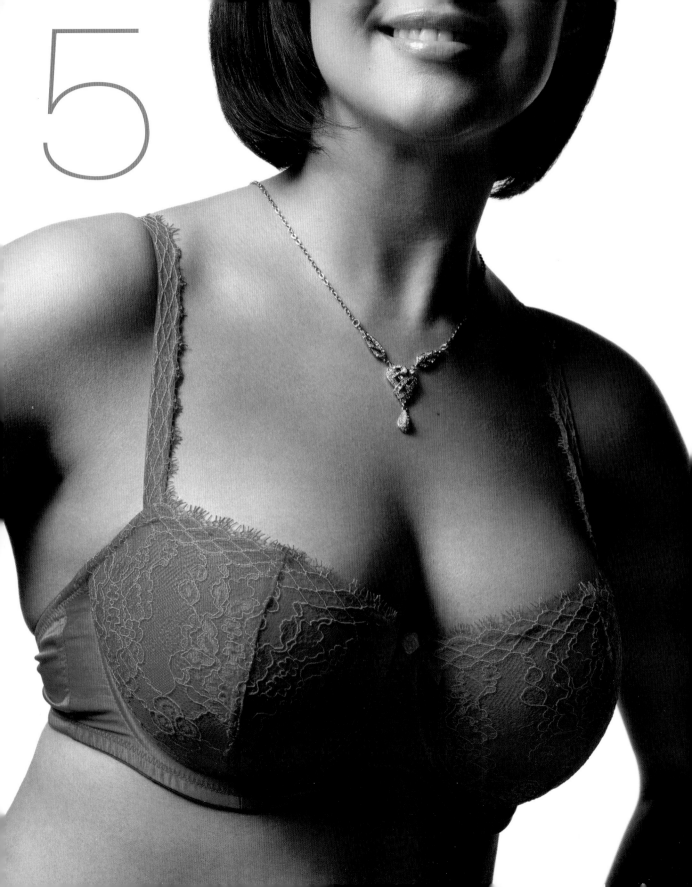

5

Big Bust

AKA

saggy boobs, girlfriends, bazooms, the twins, puppies, the girls, mammaries, maracas, jugs, melons, headlights, knockers, tatas

YOU KNOW YOU HAVE IT WHEN...

You wear an empire top and everyone assumes you're pregnant... You look down and can't see your feet... You can keep a cell phone in your cleavage... Your dream is to go braless in tank tops... Men seem to glance at your chest before your face.

→ This is the one chapter in which I have to admit up front that I took the "extreme" route to looking Fit Not Fat. I had breast-reduction surgery. My only regret is that I didn't do it earlier in my life, as soon as I was emotionally prepared, back in my college days. But until my cousin Lisa told me that she read about it in a magazine, I wasn't even aware that the surgery existed! When you are five feet tall, wearing a triple D, you can minimize your bust a bit, but you can't hide it. I often felt that when someone looked at me, all they could see was chest. And, with breasts that big, I never looked thin. Because I wasn't thin! I was top-heavy, plus I gained a lot of weight in my lower half because it's hard to get motivated to diet and exercise when you have to shoulder all that excess weight. I didn't realize that the reason I seemed allergic to physical fitness (I never once entered the gym during four years at college) was that I couldn't run or do aerobics without discomfort. Even doubling up on sports bras, jogging was painful. I took golf lessons one summer until the pro pulled me aside to tell me that he thought this was never going to be my game because I got in the way of myself with every swing. For a high school kid taking lessons with all her friends, this was very embarrassing! I avoided swimming because swimwear was impossible to fit. Back then, you couldn't buy different-sized tops and bottoms, so every suit that would accommodate my bosom was ginormous elsewhere.

The reason I'm telling you all this is because there are big breasts, and then there are breasts so out of proportion to your body that, for some of us, they can restrict our quality of life. If you're in the latter category like I was, you'll want to read the section Going to Extremes (see page 82). For everyone else, lifting your breasts to the proper position will make you look ten pounds thinner, and it's as quick and as easy as slipping on the right bra. And once you've found The One, know what your no-fat clothes options are so you can flaunt your assets in the most Fit Not Fat way possible. ●

for a Big Bust

→SO IT STARTS WITH THE RIGHT BRA. Then, it's all about learning how to choose clothes that show off your shape without exaggerating your size. I know you've heard this a zillion times before, but the last report I saw said that 85 percent of us are walking around in the wrong bra. And did you know that the average woman wears six or seven different bra sizes in her lifetime? (I know at least one woman who has seven different bra sizes in her drawer right now due to yo-yo dieting.) I promised you fast and easy ways to look thinner without dieting, and I can't think of an easier way to look like you've dropped down a size or two than this: Get yourself to a store where you can get bra-fitted today. Whether you're closest to a major department store such as Bloomingdale's or Nordstrom or a specialty shop like the Intimacy boutique, you usually don't need an appointment to get fitted. (Stop in the lingerie department first so you can do your other shopping instead of wasting time if they tell you to come back in a half hour.) If you've gained or lost five to ten pounds, been pregnant, changed your fitness regimen, had breast surgery (including implants), or haven't been fitted since high school, a new size bra may be all you need to look Fit

Not Fat, which is why every "Look Ten Years Younger" TV makeover I do starts off with a new bra!

The dress-thinner strategy here involves creating as much space as possible between your waist and chest. I must repeat this here and highlight it.

> The dress-thinner strategy here involves creating as much space as possible between your waist and chest.

Why? Because a longer torso will make you look leaner. Got it? You need a bra that can lift your breasts up and off the rib cage. If you hoist your bust up, you'll be exposing the space beneath your bra band, elongating your midriff, and showing off a few extra inches of upper torso. Just think about it: If your boobs are resting on top of your belly button, you'll miss out on having this thin spot on your body.

How far up do they need to be? You're up enough if (in your bra) your nipples are equidistant from the top of your shoulder to your elbow, no lower. Keep in mind: You want a full-coverage bra here, one

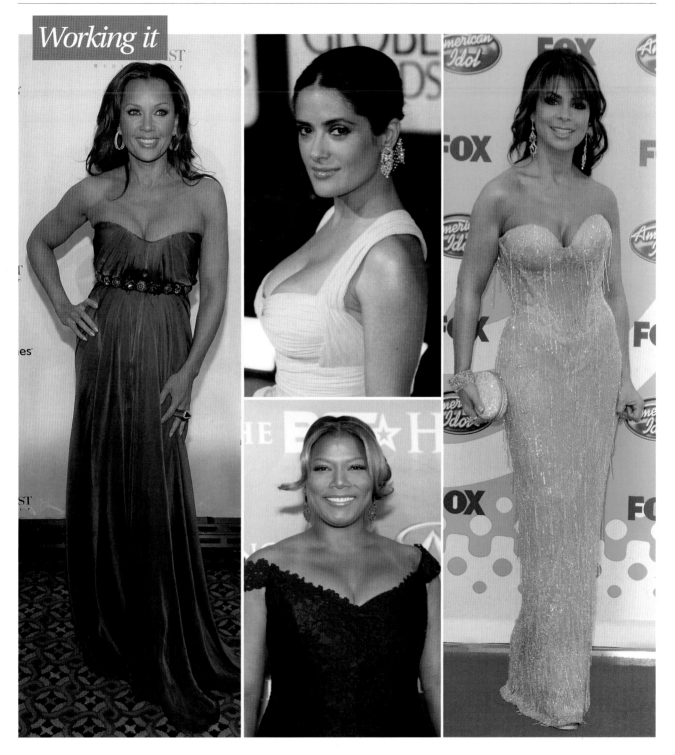

Working it

Join this support group. They know from great bras.

Clockwise from left: VANESSA WILLIAMS, SALMA HAYEK, PAULA ABDUL, QUEEN LATIFAH

that covers your entire breast—no demis, no pushups. They'll do nothing to help you and will only make you look chestier and saggier than you are. You have to be demanding here—not all full-coverage bras are created equal, and some that are soft and stretchy won't provide all the leverage and control you need. Case in point: the Spanx Bra-llelujah! I love this bra for wearing around the house, but does it provide the absolute best lift-off when I need to be up, up, up? No, no, no. That's why you need a wardrobe of bras for different situations. And don't settle when you're looking for uplift.

BE PICKY WHEN SHOPPING FOR A BRA
BE PICKY ABOUT SIZING
Some of us are so independent that we take pride in trying to figure out everything on our own. A very admirable trait, but not when it includes Googling "how to determine bra size." Don't bother whipping out a tape measure and calculator, because those tables are not reliable, and this isn't something you can afford to guess at. A professional bra-fitter can best determine whether you, like most women, are wearing a band too big and cups too small. Try a bra first on the loosest hook—not the tightest—because you want the flexibility to tighten the bra at a later date when every-

day wear causes it to stretch. It's a smart way to extend the shelf life of your investment.

Larger-size women are finally starting to get the assortment they deserve from brands such as Wacoal, Fantasie, Panache, and Chantelle, who offer gorgeous bras lavished with lace, color, and details every bit as feminine and sexy as size A's. Some brands now go up to KK and L.

Don't get hung up on a letter. Did you know that, unfortunately, there is no standardization of cup sizes? Not between countries, not between brands within the same country, and not even in styles within the same brand. You might be a DD in one style and an E in another from the same manufacturer! So if you order bras internationally online, you have to look at the size charts, because a US 34DDD is a UK 34E and a French 90F.

BE PICKY ABOUT CONSTRUCTION
If you have a healthy, full bust, rather than treat it as a curse, appreciate it! It's why all those women, who have made breast augmentation the most popular plastic surgery (in 2008, according to American Society for Aesthetic Plastic Surgery), go under the knife. Your best everyday bra will be a full-coverage bra. Whether you choose molded or seamed depends on your size; for larger sizes, the fit

is better in a seamed bra, says Susan Nethero, owner of the Intimacy boutiques.

A molded bra. I'm crazy about these seamless, preformed, heat-molded cups because you can get a high, firm, rounded shape and great separation without a stiff feeling. Even though it's been around a while, I still love Le Mystere Dream Tisha Bra, because it gives extra support under fitted clothes and light fabrics (without feeling like you're wearing a mattress). If your current molded bras leave your breasts squished, create a uni-boob, or make your bosom spill over at the sides, you need to up the cup. A molded bra can provide the lift and separation you need to avoid a uni-boob look. (When you have time on your hands, walking down the street or at the airport, see how many uni-boobs you can spot. You won't have enough fingers to count!)

A seamed bra that's contoured, cut, and sewn for engineered lift. This is best for very big and saggy breasts. By directing breast tissue toward the center of the bra, a seamed bra provides extra coverage and shaping and gives maximum compression and lift. Wacoal's Romantic Encounters style is an example of a seamed bra. Don't let wide back bands deter you. More heavy lifting is done in the band than → *continued on page 79*

WHY YOUR BREASTS ARE
GETTING BIGGER

It may surprise you to know that the most popular bra size sold in the United States by Wacoal has ballooned from 34B to 36DD in ten years—and it's not due to implants, according to Liz Smith, director of retail services at Wacoal America. "Yes, the average size ten years ago was a 34B, but who knows how accurate that was, since most women didn't get fitted and just wore the same size year after year, probably the same bra size since high school," says Smith. "Part of it is we're getting bigger, we're gaining weight, and bigger breasts are part of the package." To accommodate our growth spurt, bra-fitting boutique Intimacy, which has stores across the country, now stocks up to a size K!

With as little as a five-pound weight gain, our breasts, which consist mostly of fat, can get fatter. With menopause, women who were small-busted are happy to spring serious breasts, while women who were already endowed don't welcome being super-sized. Call this phenomenon part of nature's Fat Redistribution Program! That's the best explanation I've heard on the subject, and it comes from Dr. Pamela Peeke: "Fat gets redistributed as we age, and it causes many women, even slender women, to go up a cup. A lot of fat settles in the breast and below the bra line," she tells us, referring to back fat.

And then there's sag: Sag is going to get most of us sooner or later, as it's not easy to defy gravity. Ligaments stretch, the skin loses elasticity, and if you lose weight in your breasts, that deflation could result in longer breasts that droop like post-party balloons. (What? You thought you were the only one?) If your breasts are heading south toward your waistline, the right bra, as I've said before, is your low-maintenance breast-lift. You may feel more comfortable going braless in your own home, but you're only going to encourage the fried-egg look with increased loss of elasticity. Better you should find a bra so super-comfy that you'll want to sleep in it! (See Brilliant Buys, Spanx Bra-llelujah!, page 84).

What you can do about it: Eat healthy food and exercise, of course, but what else is new? Health advocates concerned about America's obesity are constantly telling us to reduce the amount of artificial additives in our foods. Dr. Peeke agrees: "If you don't watch what you eat, your breasts will suffer the impact of poor nutrition, and that will be exacerbated by lack of exercise." The cold, hard truth is that if you choose to eat healthy foods instead of a lot of processed junk food, and remove excess weight through diet and exercise, your breasts will downsize maybe a cup size or two, which can make a huge difference in how your clothes fit. Of course, if you start serious weight training, your bra-band size might increase as the muscles lying under the breast firm up. Ideally, you want to lose volume in the breast and develop your chest muscles to firm up support beneath the breast, so you keep those babies up there.

HIGH FAT *vs.* NO FAT

→ A big bosom adds width to the upper body and, frankly, it's easier to handle if you're tall and busty. But many women with big chests are short and buxom and are fighting the tendency to look boxy in their clothes. When it comes to jackets, for example, the less frou-frou front and center the better.

HIGH FAT:
A too-wide belt chops you up in two pieces. A tight, safari jacket with patch pockets that pull across the bust makes you look all-chest.

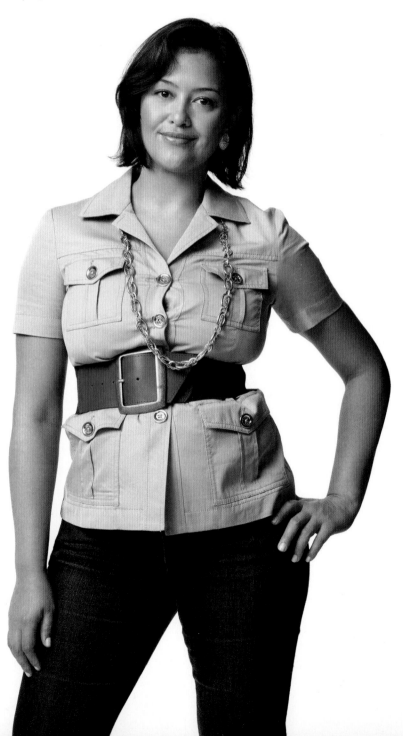

HOW FAST CAN YOU GIVE THESE AWAY?

HIGH FAT

× Baby doll dresses

× Bustiers

× Double-breasted jackets, coats

× Long necklaces and pendants that dangle near the boobs

× Patch pocket shirts, jackets

× Strapless dresses

× Wide belts at the waist

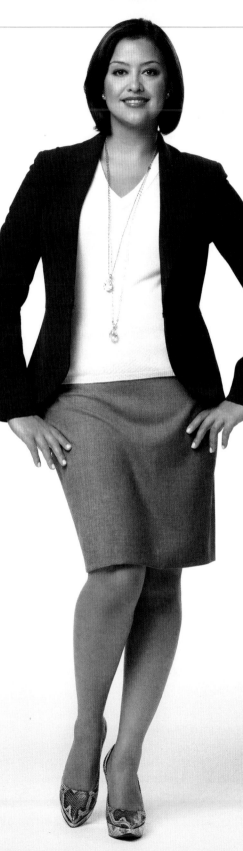

NO FAT:
A tailored jacket that's nipped in at the waist over a long V-neck top with lengthy pendants draws attention south of the bustline.

YOU CAN'T HAVE TOO MANY OF THESE!

NO FAT

√ Fitted single-breasted suits with hip-length jackets

√ Hip belts

√ One-shoulder dresses

√ Ruched and draped jersey tops

√ Sheath dresses with V-necks

√ Tunics with split neckline and decorative beading

√ V-neck sweaters and cardigans

10 THINGS THAT MAKE YOU LOOK FAT WITH A *Big Bust*

1. **Patch pockets over the breasts** add extra padding and provide a target for attention just where you don't need it. Patch flap pockets with buttons are disastrous. This includes safari jackets, which we love but don't love us back.

2. **Tucking in tops** is one of the worst things you can do. It shortens your torso and makes a big chest look bigger than it has to. But you already know that. If you're short waisted to start, tucking in leaves you with no midriff at all. Remember that it's all about elongating the midriff.

3. **Long necklaces that end below the bust** and dangle mid-air like rock climbers emphasize the ledge of your bosom and have an old-fashioned granny look. Ditto: An eyeglass chain resting on your chest is not a slimming look since it invariably loops itself around a boob. Stick your glasses on your head or nose.

4. **Tightness across the chest.** In fitted sweaters, buy the next size. Ditto, buttoned-up shirts or cardigans that crease horizontally and gape at buttonholes to reveal your bra.

5. **Turtlenecks,** because they close you in and call attention to the widest, fullest area between your chin and waist—your chest.

6. **Excessive cleavage, pushed-together boobs.** Skip bustiers, pushup, and balcony bras.

7. **Tight T-shirts.** White ones magnify your chest size. Shirts that express statements expand like a billboard.

8. **Strapless gowns, tops and swimsuits** (more in Chapter 12). They can leave you droopy and tugging upward for more support.

9. **Across-the-body messenger or shoulder bag.** The strap emphasizes breasts and traps them in a frame.

10. **Bulky jackets and sweaters.** Tough leather motorcycle jackets, blousons, bombers, stiff-pocketed jean jackets, and big fisherman's sweaters all make you look broader, tougher, and bigger.

in the straps. In fact, your bra should stay up and in place without the help of straps pulling to the max. If you get red indentations on your shoulders, you're asking too much of your straps. The bra should sit snugly around your rib cage and not creep up, creating rolls of skin.

A minimizer bra would seem like a no-brainer for someone who wants to look smaller. But while a minimizer can be useful when you don't want to worry about pulling and gaps between the buttons on buttoned-up shirts, jackets, and cardigans, be aware that you are trading shape for compression. For years, I wore minimizers because I cared more about being smaller than about the fact that I was mashing myself into a mass that looked like four breasts. Yes, I looked flatter, but I also had an overall weird, chunky look, particularly since I had a huge chest and short torso. Think about it: If the flesh isn't going up and out, it has to go somewhere, and where it's going is out to the sides and down. Susan Nethero of Intimacy doesn't believe in minimizers and doesn't even buy them for her boutiques. "They tend to spread the breast across the body and make a person look thicker and wide," she says. Who wants that? "Compression is a poor way to pro-

vide support and it will cause you to lose firmness. The best technique for minimizing a full bust is to find bra styles that bring the bust line within the body frame and give additional lift, which will make you look thinner in a minute."

Look around at any party and there are always women who play the breast card, exposing too much bosom, especially at a black-tie business affair. They always make every other woman feel uncomfortable. Men, too, feel awkward because they don't know where to look. Why would you want everyone staring at your chest when they could be staring at your face? If you want to play it sultry for the evening, body-hugging—not flesh-revealing—is the classier way to go. If you can't help yourself, and decide to take the plunge for a black-tie event, make sure the neckline of your gown is a V no deeper than your usual bra dip, covering three-quarters of your breasts. You always want to look elegant, not desperate, no matter what your size.

BE PICKY ABOUT WHAT BRA YOU WEAR UNDER WHAT OUTFIT

Your bra has to work with your body and your outfit, and the wrong bra can make you look bustier—and heavier. For example, a sexy lace pushup bra is not going to help you if you're a 36E and wearing a silky blouse. The lace will show through and buttons will pull as your bosom is pushed up and out. Choose a bra for support first, eye appeal second. Fancy bras can leave lumps, bumps, and bulges under thin knits, tees, sweaters and light fabrics and make you look sloppy when you need to look totally pulled together and Fit Not Fat. Granted, supportive bras are not as pretty, but a seamless T-shirt bra with a molded cup will prevent show-thru on light fabrics, matte jerseys, tees, and fine-knit sweaters.

Obviously, everyone's lifestyle doesn't require every type of bra. One of the makeovers I did on the *Oprah* show was on a busy mom who only owned one bra—a sports bra. I felt so badly for her! Needless to say, the first order of business was getting her fitted for a basic everyday T-shirt bra, because you don't have

- A T-shirt bra should be seamless, and is often molded, to give you smooth lift and coverage under fitted, light clothing.

- A structured bra with seams works well under tailored shirts and jackets. It shapes you, but it won't give you a pointy retro look.

- A racerback bra is for halter-style sleeveless tops and dresses that cut in at the neck and shoulders.

- A strapless bra is what you need for those stylish off-the-shoulder, one-shoulder, and strapless tops and dresses.

- A deep V-bra lets you take the dive you need without showing your bra in V-neck sweaters, dresses, and wraps.

- A sports bra keeps your breasts close to your body under stretchy nylon workout tops. Your ligaments and tissue need a supportive frame. You want to avoid stretch marks, commonly a result of heavy breasts dealing with motion and gravity.

- A fancy sexy bra should be considered only for intimate moments, as they usually don't offer enough support under clothes . . . then again, you may not be wearing it under clothes.

to sacrifice shape for comfort. But if the goal is to look fit, firm, and fashionable, you want to be prepared and have the right type of bra sitting in your drawer, so when getting dressed for a party, interview, wedding, whatever, there is no need for last-minute panic if your clothing requires a special bra. So choose what you need from this list at left. And, once you find your perfect everyday bra, you may want to buy three—two nudes and a black or two blacks and one nude, depending on your wardrobe. You don't need a white bra, nude looks better under white than white.

SHOWING YOUR SHAPE WITHOUT INCREASING YOUR SIZE

Now that you know everything about finding the right bra, how best to dress it? I'm not going to tell you to wear black and only black. Why? Because you already know that black optically diminishes size better than any other color. And because an exclusively black wardrobe is depressing . . . chic,

but depressing. But underneath jackets and cardigans, you need a wardrobe of dark tees, camisoles, tanks, and sweaters as standard layering pieces.

Many of us get in a rut and only think black, but anything that's dark will be slimmer than light. So consider layering pieces in navy, charcoal, brown, eggplant, forest green, and burgundy, too. They should be pieces that you look and feel great in, because you will depend on them and wear them often. Tailored fitted jackets and blazers are the next style sanctuary for women with generous chests. Their sharp lines add welcome angularity to a rounded upper body. Stay classic and wear them over fitted tees or a camisole or trend them up with draped or layered pieces. And because you're big busted, you need to know that overexposing your breasts and showing cleavage in deep dip necklines is tacky—even if you're getting an Oscar! ●

If the goal is to look fit, firm, and fashionable, you want to be prepared and have the right type of bra sitting in your drawer, so when getting dressed for a party, interview, wedding, whatever, there is no need for last-minute panic if your clothing requires a special bra.

Thinner by Tonight!

INSTANT GRATIFICATION

Put on your brand-new, perfect-fitting bra.
Your chest just got a makeover.

Show a bit of skin (not deep cleavage) with a V neckline.
The open inverted triangle creates a higher horizontal focal point up and away from the one your boobs naturally create and gives you a longer, slimmer upper body.

Create a slim zone
just beneath your bosom with a raised waist or empire top that defines the slimmer rib cage just under your bra. Large, shapeless tops just make you look big and bulky all over.

Slip on a slimming jacket.
The straight lines, narrow V, and slim lapels of a blazer counteract excess curves with a crisp shape.

Layer your way slim.
Sandwich long body-skimming tanks or shaper camisoles between your bra and relaxed A-shape tees or sweaters. The buffer layer prevents clothes from sticking to curves and looks stylishly hip.

Lower your waist to create more midriff space by wearing a belt lower on the top of the hip. Try this on tops worn out over jeans or sheath dresses and shifts. Your boobs will seem to float higher.

Wear heels.
Adding inches to your legs evens out your body proportions. Trust me, it will make your chest appear more in proportion and less prominent.

Keep skirts around knee-length give or take an inch. Going too short makes you look top-heavy. Leave the micro-minis to ballerina bodies and teens.

De-emphasize your bosom with reversed color strategy.
Switch the usual tactic and wear dark on top, light on bottom. A black tee and white jeans might be your new dress-slim weekend uniform. This is a trick from my friends in Miami who live in white pants!

Take a yoga or Pilates class or stretch or get a massage to lose the hunched-over look.
Ease the tension in the shoulders and neck that can make busty women look caved-in and inches shorter. Yes, a heavy load on your chest can cause muscle strain, so be kind to yourself, and get rid of the rock-hard tension. Just keep your shoulders back, and you will immediately look leaner!

BIG BUST SOLUTIONS

• **WEAR DRESSES RATHER THAN SEPARATE TOPS AND BOTTOMS.** If you're short and bosomy, you don't have much room between the neck and waist, so pieces crunch your mid-riff space. Dresses help stretch your torso and body visually while they de-emphasize the top.

• **KEEP BELTS LOW ON THE WAIST** (loose rather than snug) so they dip in front, and blouse your dress by pulling it out a bit to soften the shape. If your dress comes with a belt, remove the loops. Watch belt size: too wide and it will be resting on your boobs. (If your belts need another hole or two, bring them to a shoemaker or a hammer/nail will do. If your belts need shortening, bring them in also as excess belt length looped around is fattening.)

• **DUPLICATE NECKLINES WHEN LAYERING TO KEEP IT SIMPLE.** A deep V sweater over a soft shirt that is unbuttoned to a low V works; a shallow scoop-neck sweater over a shallow scoop-neck tank works, too.

• If you're busty and short with a wide derriere, SKIP CROPPED JACKETS BECAUSE THEY'LL ONLY EXAGGERATE YOUR WIDTH, and pass up long jackets because they'll make your legs seem super-short. Choose semi-fitted mid-hip jackets.

• Hourglass figures with full tops and bottoms can look great in the GRACEFUL FOLDS OF A SOFT JERSEY WRAP DRESS that plays up a narrow waist and creates definition between the two more generous body zones.

Going to Extremes: *Breast Surgery*

If you are financially and emotionally prepared, and feel that your breasts are truly out of sync with the rest of your body, surgery is an option. When bra shopping is a nightmare, you can't wear the clothes you want, you feel inhibited with your significant other, and doing sports or appearing in a swimsuit makes you self-conscious, a breast reduction or lift could really change your life.

BREAST-REDUCTION SURGERY. If your breasts are so heavy you can't remember a time when your bra straps weren't digging into your shoulders and leaving big red grooves, a reduction could relieve the strain of carrying around that extra four pounds (about two pounds a breast). A lift is a standard part of a reduction because you're dealing with removal of tissue, fat, and skin, both size and sag. Your bra band size may not change at all; it's your cup that sees the difference. This is serious surgery and not to be taken lightly, as complications can arise.

A BREAST LIFT. A breast lift will reposition saggy nipples that have drooped downward pointing to your waist, but the breasts themselves stay the same size. If your nipples have sagged below the breast crease, and your boobs look long and tubular, the nipple can be lifted and the breast reshaped with a mastopexy. Implants alone will not raise your nipples higher; they just increase the size of your breasts. If you have a generous C cup that's hanging, an implant could, in

IF YOU'RE SIZE 14 & UP...

• WEAR JACKETS AND TOPS THAT REACH THE HIPBONE IN LENGTH to balance excess width at the bust; cropped jackets are not best for you.

• KEEP NECKLINES SIMPLE AND FREE OF FRILLS. The broader and bigger your chest and overall proportions, the less fussy your necklines should be. Skip the frou-frou fancy collars. Abby Z., a New York City stylist and designer for larger sizes, says, "Make all your tops as V-neck as possible; it's the most flattering neckline for a large bust."

• MINIMIZE BULKY LAYERING WITH THIN, FLAT FABRICS THAT HAVE "SLIP." A crisp button-down shirt under a ribbed and cabled cotton sweater will add pounds; a soft silk blouse under a flat-knit fine-gauge sweater subtracts them.

• KEEP JACKET DETAILS ON THE QUIET SIDE. Be sure buttons are small and color toned to the garment. Watch the width of lapels; oversized is fattening. Nothing should scream out at you.

fact, increase the sag! Very large nipples that protrude over the areola are sometimes a result of breast-feeding, and these can be trimmed down, too, at the same time. You may experience loss of feeling or change of color in the nipples.

BREAST IMPLANTS. Augmentation surpassed liposuction for the first time in 2008 as the most popular cosmetic surgery, though it's not on the rise. According to the American Society of Aesthetic Plastic Surgery, there were 355,671 breast implants in 2008, down from 399,440 in 2007. Why discuss implants in a chapter about already-too-big breasts? There are women who opt for breast implants to balance weight gain in the lower body—fuzzy logic, to be sure, as the overall goal is to look smaller, not bigger. Women who get implants will undoubtedly find fashion as challenging as it is for their naturally large sisters, as the same big-bust rules apply. ●

A BUST-FRIENDLY GUIDE TO NECKLINES

Ballet
A shallow scoop, think leotard, looks elegant and classic.

Cowl-draped
Bares neck and gracefully camouflages

Faux Wrap
Pre-styled crossover for subtle camouflage and shaping

Halter
A high-neck/back shell with deeply cutaway armholes

Henley
Round neck, button placket tee worn open reveals skin

Polo
Classic collar and button placket worn open makes a small V

Ruched
A scoop or ballet neck with gathered fabric

Scoop
Sculpts and bares collarbones; good for boobs with no sag

Square
Refocuses attention above breasts and spares cleavage

Tie-neck
Tied low or high grabs attention away from bosom

V
Inverts the bustline-to-neck triangle to rebalance proportions

BRILLIANT BUYS

BEST EVERYDAY FULL COVERAGE BRA

Le Mystere Tech Fit Bra, style 954, 32–38 B–E, $69; Bloomingdale's, bloomingdales.com. Lightweight, well-designed to cover the entire breast so it doesn't leave you with major boob spillage, a.k.a. four boobs.

BEST EVERYDAY BRA FOR A RANGE OF SKIN TONES

MySkins T-shirt Bra, 32A–38D, $60; myskins.com. Pretty, scalloped, seamless bra that comes in 20 skin tones.

BEST FEMININE BRAS FOR BIG BUSTS

Le Mystere Baroque Tisha Bra, style 9966, 32–42, C–G, $76; herroom.com. A prettier T-shirt bra that supports full cups.

BEST MINIMIZERS

Le Mystere Dream Minimizer Bra, style 311, 32–42, C–G, $62; Dillard's, barenecessities .com. Super soft and comfortable while still supportive.

Wacoal SlimLine Seamless Minimizer, style 85154, 34C–40DDD, $65; Nordstrom, barenecessities.com. Reduces your bust up to one full inch.

Lilyette Plunge Into Comfort Minimizer Bra, style 904, $32; barenecessities.com. A cushioned underwire, a contemporary bare look, and a wide plunge neck so it's great for V-necklines.

BEST FOR BACK FAT

Spanx Bra-llelujah! Underwire Contour Bra, style 216, 32–36 A, 32–38 B–D, 40–42 C–D, 32–42 DD, $62; Bloomingdale's, spanx.com. It's super comfortable and has more support for bigger busts than the original all-hosiery, wireless Bra-llelujah. Also available in non-padded and racerback styles.

Assets Brilliant Bra, up to 38D, $32; Target, target.com. A back fat–busting bra that fastens in the front, much like the Bra-llelujah! from Spanx

Shapeez Unbelievabra The Shortee, XS A–1XDD, $75; Van Mauer, shapeez.com.

DON'T WASTE A PENNY ON . . .

Bust-firming treatments that claim to lift your bosom with natural firmers like wheat proteins and horse chestnut extract. You might get silkier skin, but it takes more than a topical cream to get your boobs back to perky. Better to spend the cash on a good supportive bra.

Vows *for the* Big Busted

- ☐ **I WILL** get bra-fitted once a year.

- ☐ **I WILL** rid my lingerie drawer of old stretched out bras and remember that bras don't retain shape forever —only 100 washings!

- ☐ **I WILL** treat my new bras with TLC—and wash by hand, not throw them into the washing machine, and worse, the dryer.

- ☐ **I WILL** look through my closet and figure out the kinds of bras I need—and go shopping before I need them.

- ☐ **I WILL NOT** dangle necklaces off the cliff of my chest.

- ☐ **I WILL** wear a camisole under wrap dresses and not reveal excessive cleavage.

- ☐ **I WILL NOT** flaunt big saggy boobs with low-cut cleavage at parties.

- ☐ **I WILL** ease shoulder tension and back strain with a massage treat at a day spa or stretching classes.

DON'T YOU DARE…

Exercise braless. It's an open invitation to sag!

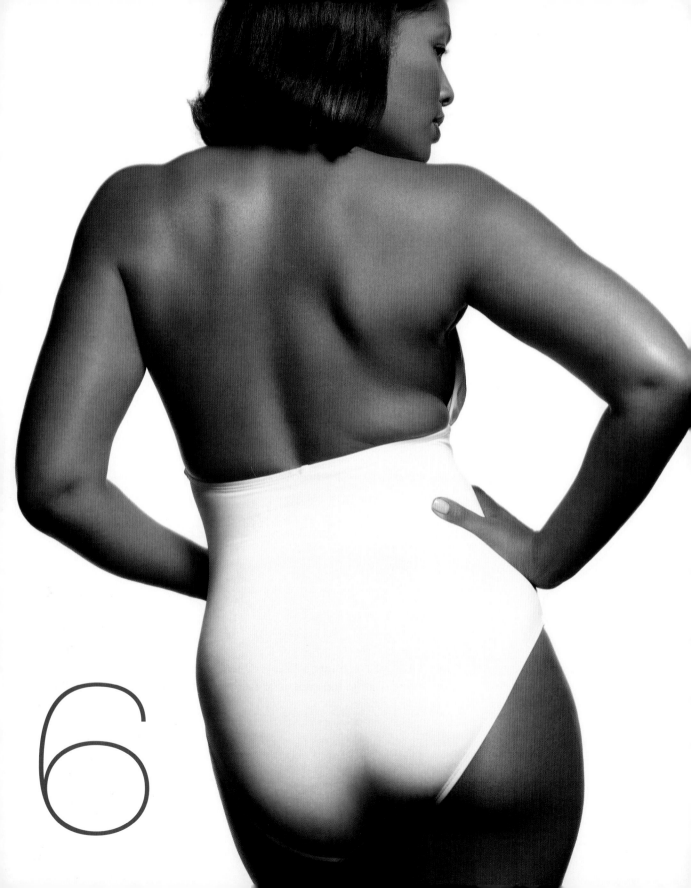

6

Muffin Top + Back Fat

AKA

love handles, mushroom effect, spare tire, tummy overhang, stomach spillage, midriff bulge, split muffin, back boobs, bra roll, sofa-back, dolphin-back

YOU KNOW YOU HAVE IT WHEN. . .

Your flesh balloons over the waistband of your jeans... You can pinch way more than an inch all around your middle... You wear a jacket or cardigan for protection... You avoid friendly hugs... You're embarrassed to get a massage... Your bras feel better on the last hook... Stretch tees with Lycra® make you worry.

→ Remember when jeans and a tee were the easiest, most comfortable things to wear? But as jeans dipped to super-low-rise at the same time the tight short top became fashion, women of a certain age discovered two new unwelcome body parts: muffin top and back fat. Something tells me that if you're reading this, you don't need definitions, but it's fun to know that "muffin top" was first used as Aussie slang in 2003 and then popularized on *Kath and Kim*, a hit show on Australian TV (which obviously lost something in its U.S. translation!). In 2006, it was named new word of the year in Aussieland and has become part of the lexicon as the perfect descriptor for the flesh that blobs over our waistbands, so reminiscent of a muffin spilling out of its paper cup. In an episode of *30 Rock*, Jane Krakowski's Jenna Maroney records a song called "Muffin Top," which becomes a chart topper in Israel and Belgium!

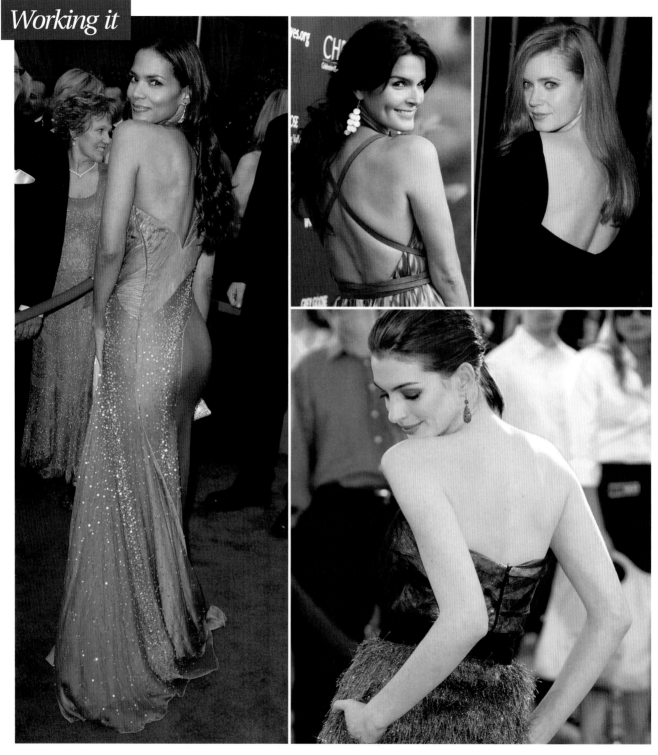

Watching their own backs.
Clockwise from left: HALLE BERRY, ANGIE HARMON, AMY ADAMS, ANNE HATHAWAY

"Back fat," those fleshy cutlets popping out above and below the back of the bra, which look like you've sprouted back boobs, is an expression that has also come into its own, with a bra dedicated to eradicating those unsightly bumps and bulges (Spanx Bra-llelujah!). Some also call muffin top from the rear view back has yet coined a word for the fleshy upper roll that seeps out from under the bra band in front—the roll above the stomach that used to be called Midriff Bulge before we started getting really specific and naming our rolls—let's refer to it as the opposite of back fat: front fat.

As women, we joke among our who are in great shape look in the mirror with shock and horror, realizing that they now have four breasts, and one is popping out under each armpit. It's a redistribution of fat, and it begins to happen to the mass majority of women between the ages of forty-five and fifty-two. During that time, two extra breasts,

WHAT ELSE CAN YOU DO ABOUT THOSE ROLLS?

Stop eating so much! You can ab crunch, you can oblique twist, you can row, you can work your core. But you have to cut your daily intake of calories, too, because you need to eliminate that layer of fat that covers your abdominal muscles. This is something we don't want to hear, but hear it we must, as our health, too, is at risk. "Women are just plain eating too much," says Dr. Pamela Peeke. "At fifty-two, you can't eat the way you did at thirty and at forty, you can't eat like you did in college at twenty cramming for exams. You keep eating like you're twenty and you're going to pay for it.

"As you age," she continues, "you have to eat less and eat smarter, too, and occasionally treat yourself to something wonderful." Dr. Peeke treats herself to one gourmet oatmeal raisin cookie, not an entire sleeve of Oreos as she once did in college. "Just like you have to put thought into what you wear, you have to put thought and value into what you eat," she says. Woman who do that, look like it. "The quality of your food is reflected in how you look. Women say to me all the time, 'But I never had to pay attention to what I ate before' and I say, 'You were never forty-five before, either. The game has changed, and you are a different biological specimen and have different needs. Honor your body, and be good to yourself.'" Amen.

fat. So that we're crystal clear here, back fat is only the roll that pops out of the bra band in the back, and muffin top from the rear view is muffin top from the rear view. (I don't really love the term "split muffin," which is used to describe a muffin top when you're bending down in low-rise jeans, do you?) And, since no one selves about these extra bulges encircling our middle, but trying to dress them is where the laughter stops and the frustration begins.

Muffin tops are democratic. You can wear a size 27 jean and have muffin top. They tend to crop up most often in midlife. According to Dr. Pamela Peeke, "Even women belly fat, and back fat will occur in a lot of women. Make sure you're getting appropriate cardio along with excellent nutrition. It will minimize any back issue that you have."

Now that we know what we're talking about, let's divide and conquer. ●

HIGH FAT *vs.* NO FAT

→ A short, snug T-shirt paired with low-slung pants is a recipe for a high fat look. Jeans should be slightly higher rise, nine inches is perfect, not so high as to be "mom jeans" and not as deep-dipping as teen jeans. Say good-bye to tight cropped tops unless you wear a visible bodysuit underneath. At right, a control camisole smoothes away back fat and bra bunching.

....

HIGH FAT:
This light colored T-shirt is so tight that it's bunching up, creating back fat, VVB (Visible Bra Band) and muffin top. No woman wants this kind of exposure.

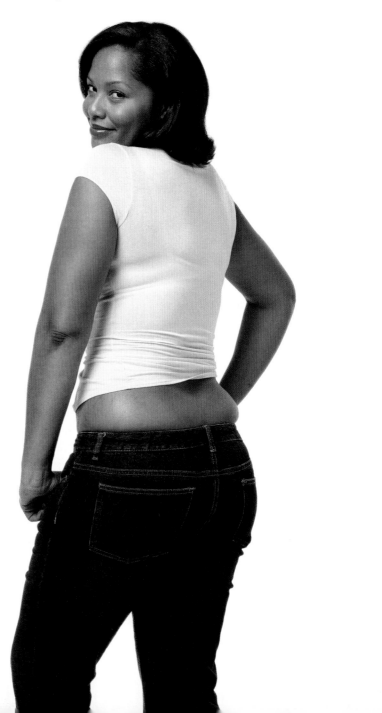

HOW FAST CAN YOU GIVE THESE AWAY?

HIGH FAT

Muffin Top

× Body-hugging knits

× Bolero jackets

× Cropped tees

× Hipster pants

Back Fat

× Clingy, fine-gauge sweaters

× Flimsy slip dresses

× Horizontal-stripe anything on top

× Strapless dresses, tops

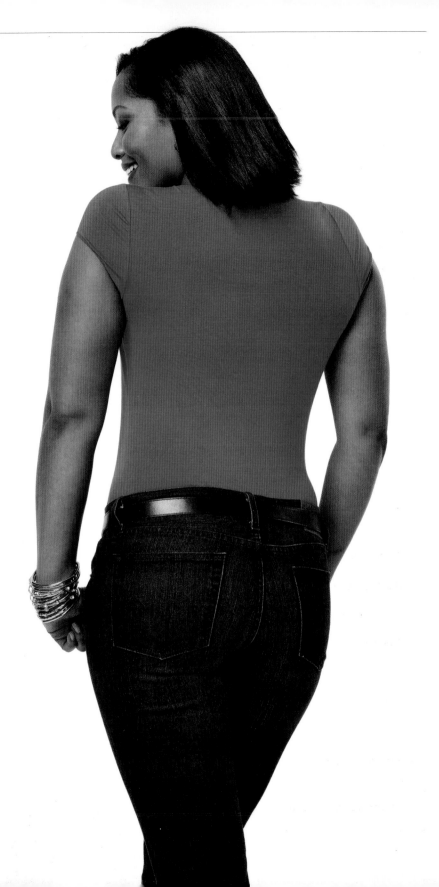

NO FAT:
This is the same T-shirt in a darker color and larger size! The longer T is tucked into higher-waisted jeans and safely secured with a belt.

YOU CAN'T HAVE TOO MANY OF THESE!

NO FAT

Muffin Top

√ Blouson blouses

√ Crisp cotton tunics

√ Print tops and dresses

√ Structured sheath dresses

Back Fat

√ A-shape tees and tops

√ Cardigans, from classic to grandpa

√ Classic-fit cashmeres in V-necks, boats, and wide scoops

√ Draped or shirred tops

Thinner by Tonight!

Wear a dress.

The simplest solution is to avoid separate tops and bottoms. But of course make that dress a raised-waist or empire V-neck or a structured sheath, not a tight knit!

Add a boyfriend cardigan or fitted jacket

as a top layer to camouflage visible love handles at the sides. It cleans up your contours instantly for a lean, trim look.

Show your arms.

If you have toned arms, go sleeveless in a dark, loose top. The illusion of an athletic upper body, shoulder to waist, is what will register.

Wear a silky blouse

that slides and skims elegantly over curves, rather than clinging to them like a sweater.

Add a vest.

Man-tailored vests over a crisp, white shirt and pants makes for a cool downtown look, while a fur or faux fur vest looks Aspen-y.

Choose a print in a swirling pattern, dots, floral, or paisley to camouflage.

Skip geometrics that tend to highlight the difference between flat and rounded body spots.

Sit up straight, like your mother told you to.

When you slouch or relax into a C-curve, your midriff compresses and flab practically ripples. Get in the habit when you're at the computer and it will become second nature in public.

Wear a camisole with an

attention-getting necklace or a ruffle-front tuxedo shirt under an open blazer. All focus will be on the center of your body.

A lace-trimmed silk or satin camisole under a

potentially bulge-making top, sweater, or dress. This stylist trick from Abby Z. works especially well when a peek of the lace shows. The slippery fabric will prevent the top from sticking to your skin.

Sling a jeweled or sequin cardigan over all your dresses and pants for evenings.

Chicer than a shawl, and newer than a pashmina, it will frame and discreetly conceal the sides of your body. Check out thrift shops, flea markets, and consignment shops for vintage finds, but contemporary designers Nanette Lepore, lisli, and Rebecca Taylor do versions of these nearly every season.

Wear a shirt open

as a jacket over a same-color base of tee or tank and pants—a very St. Tropez look. Or, an open leather motocross jacket can add an edgy look to all your clothes.

Show skin where you're

thin, but keep the flab under wraps. Visible collarbones, long and slim neck, arms, and legs all make ideal focal points to divert the eye away from your middle. This is exactly why scoop necklines were invented and why you need those new Barbie-pink patent leather heels!

MUFFIN TOP + BACK FAT SOLUTIONS

Muffin Top Solutions

- LOOK FOR SIMPLE SHIFT DRESSES WITH SMALL PRINTS TO HELP HIDE JIGGLES.

- COLLECT CARDIGANS OF VARIOUS COLORS AND FABRICS. Add an open cardigan to camouflage the sides of your body.

- WEAR HEELS WITH PANTS, SKIRTS, AND JEANS. You always need the extra length.

Back Fat Solutions

- GO UP A SIZE IN TOPS. Even a quarter inch more fabric can make a difference.

- REVERSE THE USUAL RULE AND WEAR A BLACK TOP WITH WHITE JEANS. Now a year-round look, this duo has a jet-set glamour. The black top can be anything from a black cashmere sweater to a plain Gap tee.

- LET PRINTS CONFUSE THE EYE, AND ADD SOME REAL FUN TO YOUR LOOK. This is the time to go crazy with wild, brightly colored florals and splashy, modern Pucci-like designs. Just stick to structured A-line dresses and sheaths like those by Milly, Tory Burch, Shoshanna, and Diane von Furstenberg.

Muffin Top Solutions

- CHOOSE LIGHTWEIGHT COATS AS JACKETS and look for dress/coat ensembles instead of suits and separates.

- SHIFT YOUR WAISTLINE UP TOWARD YOUR BOSOM. Raised-waist dresses and tops and empire necklines are your best choices.

- CONSIDER A CONTROL BODYSUIT for your everyday underwear to minimize layers.

Back Fat Solutions

- TREAT YOURSELF TO SOME EXOTIC DRAMA WITH CLOTHES FROM OTHER CULTURES. A beautiful sari or a salwar kameez—loose tunic with slits on the side and pants—can be discreet and distinctive evening wear.

- TONE YOUR TOP TO YOUR JACKET, BUT ADD SPICE WITH TEXTURAL DIFFERENCES—for example, a deep-violet velvet jacket and purple matte jersey top with draped neckline.

- INSTEAD OF HEAVY CABLE-KNIT SWEATERS, invest in thin long-knit scarves to wrap around your neck over loose, fine-gauge sweaters. Same cozy feel, minus the fattening effect.

Going to Extremes: *Lipo and Plastic Surgery*

LIPO ON MUFFIN TOP AND BACK FAT.
Even if you've dieted and exercised like a maniac and have a healthy weight, unwanted fat deposits and bulges can still make you cringe when you look in the mirror. Lipo can vacuum out stubborn pockets of fat such as muffin tops and back fat, but be forewarned, whether SmartLipo or standard lipo, this isn't something to be taken lightly. It's a rather rough procedure that involves significant oozing and bruising. What you need to know in this chapter is that different areas of the body react differently to lipo. If your skin is thin and loose, it can fail to tighten after lipo and look baggy. For a muffin top, the doctor has to be careful to avoid ripples, puckers, dimpling, and contour irregularities so the midriff looks balanced after the healing process, otherwise you'll have dents. The best time to do this is after you have dieted and exercised to get as close as possible to your body ideal. Some women complain that after lipo, they get fat in new areas. No one can predict where new fat will go if you gain weight again after lipo.

PLASTIC SURGERY FOR BACK FAT.
Women who have removed a massive amount of weight might be encouraged to know that there is a surgery to eliminate all that sagging skin on their back. It does leave a tell-tale scar, which is why this is not an ideal option for women who want to get rid of back fat just to wear backless dresses. ●

BRILLIANT BUYS

SHAPERS FOR MUFFIN TOP
LIGHT COMPRESSION

Spanx Skinny Britches High-Waist Short, style 930, $46; spanx.com. This is what to wear when it's hot out. Super lightweight microfiber; comes in colors.

MEDIUM COMPRESSION

Wacoal Shaping Up Long Leg Shaper, style 805161, $55; Neiman Marcus, wacoal-america.com. With an open crotch.

HEAVY DUTY COMPRESSION

TC Fine Intimates Extra Firm or Even More Hi-Waist Bike Pant, style 499, $69; bloomingdales.com.

CAMISOLES FOR BACK FAT

Flexees Instant Slimmer Firm Control Singlet, style 2556, $55; barenecessities.com. Bike short body suit with added compression in the back. Wear your own bar.

Spanx Slimplicity Open-Bust Camisole, style 309, $44; Bloomingdale's, spanx.com. Wear your own bra.

TC Fine Intimates Even More Torsette, style 4043, $56; Bloomingdale's, tcfineintimates.com. Wear your own bra.

Flexees Fat-Free Dressing Tank Top, style 3266, $38; Macy's, macys.com.

Maidenform Control It Convertible Halter Camisole, style 12404, $36; maidenform.com.

Assets Fantastic Firmers Adjustable Strap Cami, style 207, $20; Target, target.com, loveassets.com. Super soft, nice price.

DON'T WASTE A PENNY ON . . .

MESOTHERAPY

Sometimes offered at medi-spas, this is a cocktail injected under the skin that promises to "melt fat away." Three things you need to know: There is no scientific evidence that it is safe. There is no scientific evidence that it works. These under-the-skin injections for fat removal have many brand names (such as Lipodissolve) but none have been FDA-approved (as of yet). So save your money.

HOW TO *NEVER* LOOK FAT AGAIN

Vows *for* Muffin Top + Back Fat

☐ **I WILL NOT** wear hip-hugging anything.

☐ **I WILL NOT** try to squeeze into jeans that have shrunk.

☐ **I WILL NOT** put my jeans in the dryer.

☐ **I WILL NOT** wear a backless dress.

☐ **I WILL** wear control camis to hide the back fat.

☐ **I WILL** toss tops so tight that they cut and pinch.

DON'T YOU DARE . . .

Continue to wear super-low-riding jeans. There's nothing cute about a whale-tale thong hanging out!

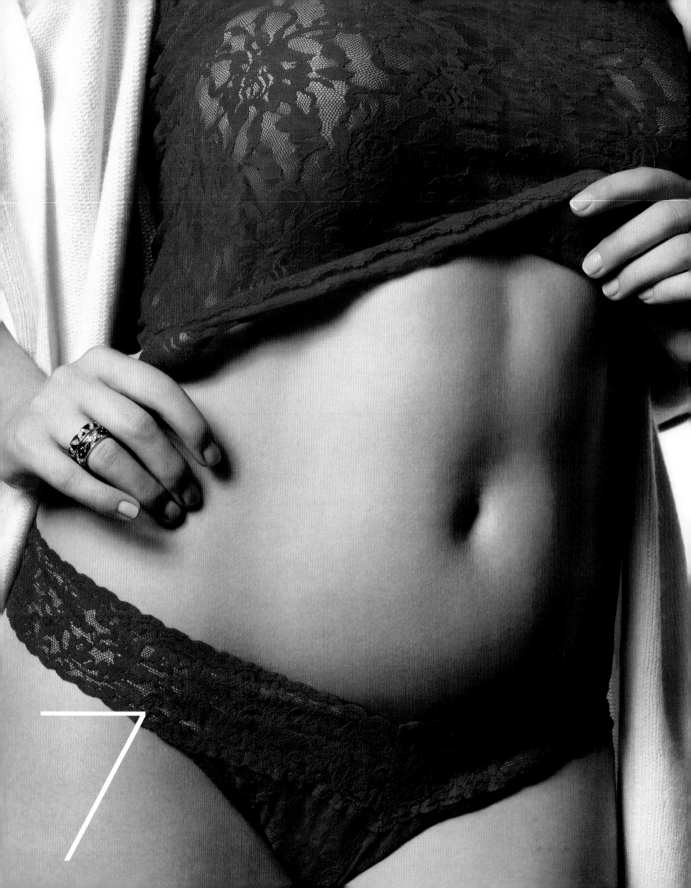

HOW TO NEVER LOOK FAT WITH A

Buddha Belly

AKA
jelly belly,
belly fat,
pot belly,
belly rolls,
menopot,
girly gut,
breadbasket,
spare tire,
thick middle,
post-baby
belly, pooch

YOU KNOW YOU HAVE IT WHEN. . .
You can't suck it in even when you try . . . Lately you prefer the missionary position . . . Sales associates have asked when the baby is due . . . Your stomach blocks your thong when you look down . . . In profile your tummy protrudes more than your chest.

→ Stand straight and pinch your skin from your belly button to where bikini underwear would start. If you can grab a roll of flab, you have a belly. Join the club. It doesn't matter if you're size 4, 14, or 20, whether you're on a diet, or whether you work out—if you're a woman of a certain age, chances are you don't have the flat tummy you once did . . . or thought was just a few crunches away!

A prominent pooch gets in the way of fashion because it's smack in the middle of your body and affects what you wear on top and bottom equally. The reason for that belly can be any number of things but is probably a combo of these: *1)* It popped out after a pregnancy or a C-section that left you with flaccid muscles, *2)* hormonal changes due to menopause have shifted fat to the tummy, *3)* you're so busy working or taking care of everyone else (or both) that you haven't take the time to exercise, *4)* you haven't cut back on your calorie consumption in recent years, or *5)* you're a woman in midlife. I have friends who do everything right, including crunches daily, and they still complain about the menopot. (Credit for this word to describe menopausal belly bulge goes to Dr. Pamela Peeke, who coined it in her book, *Body for Life for Women*.)

So what can you do about it?
Thanks to control undergarments, compression is one way to minimize the menopot; and, in fact, living in bike shorts is your easiest way to drop a size fast. For best results, you'll want to add some secret camouflage into the mix, which we'll detail throughout this chapter. Of course, losing the belly fat through weight training, crunches, aerobics, and by reducing your caloric intake is ideal. But let's be honest, it takes forever, and removing it completely, through surgery, is a major big deal. So let's do what we can to fake it, right here, right now, with clothes that practically manage your middle for you by compressing the flesh and camouflaging the evidence. And away we go. ●

YOUR DRESS-THINNER STRATEGY
for a Buddha Belly

→FOR STARTERS, YOU HAVE TO WEAR shapewear instead of regular underwear, but shapewear is just the foundation. Realize that you can't continue to dress the way you always have. Once you reach a certain age, baring the belly in low-rise jeans and cropped tops is no longer adorable. There really is no point to exposing excess flesh unless you're under thirty, a model, a dancer, or nine months pregnant posing for your pre-baby portrait. Even former belly flashers like Madonna and Cindy Crawford have adopted a more sophisticated fashion mantra. When you have a belly, you need to make your stomach recede visually by shifting proportions and tweaking details in fit, fabric, and color. Don't get nuts about this. It's just one more thing that we as women have to deal with. Ready to deal? We can do this.

HERE'S WHAT YOU NEED TO DO
SWITCH ALL YOUR UNDERWEAR TO SHAPEWEAR.
If you don't already own super-controlling bike shorts, one-piece shapers, footless panty hose, and opaque stockings, you need to stock up (see Brilliant Buys, page 112). I have a separate drawer for bike shorts, and almost every day I wrestle into a pair of high-waist bike shorts by Spanx, Lipo in a Box, TC, Wacoal, or Donna Karan. Granted, thrashing around getting these on is not a pretty sight, but the ability to lose ten pounds in one minute is well worth the struggle. I have friends who remove them only for bathing and bed. One just told me that she wishes she could sleep in them!

MANAGE YOUR MIDDLE.
Your waist is so front and center that you want to avoid making it an attention-getting target. Some fashion trends, no matter how tempting they look on celebrities, will only make you look fat. On the short list: tight knits, drawstring pants, pleated skirts.

BUY A DRESS.
Because there is no break at the center to attract your eye, a dress will immediately give your shape a sleeker line through the middle. A key strategy going forward is to buy dresses, not separates. The beauty of a dress is that there is nothing easier to slip into. You don't have to worry about what goes with what and whether or not to tuck. Not all dresses are created equal, however. The dresses that will not

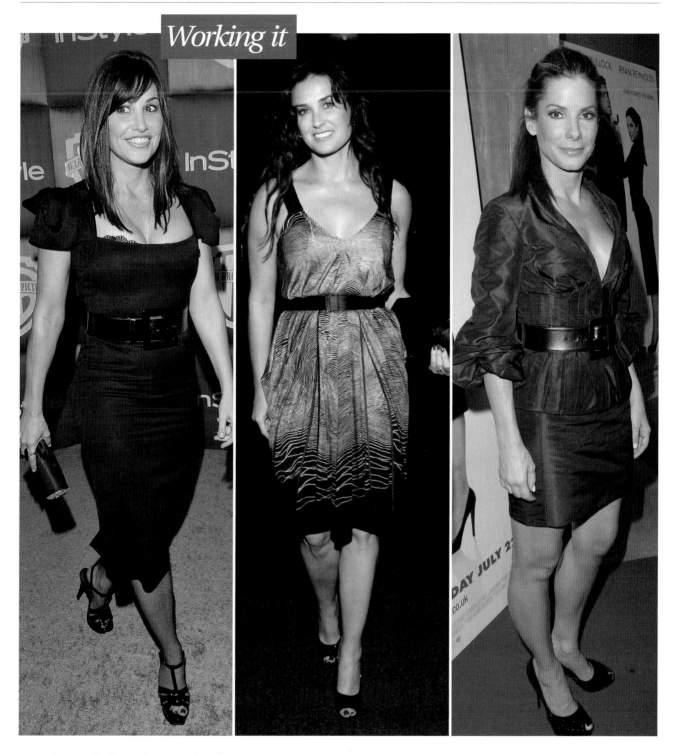

Six-pack abs or just good stylists?
GINA GERSHON, DEMI MOORE, SANDRA BULLOCK

make you look fat are the only ones we care about.

EMBRACE THE EMPIRE WAIST.
This trendy silhouette creates a higher waistline under your bust, which is probably thinner than your tummy, which it skims and hides. Because it's a fuller top, you want to keep your bottom half narrow in lean jeans, slim pants, or a pencil skirt. Find a top that isn't super voluminous, as you don't want to appear pregnant!

TWEAK THE TRENDS.
Don't follow them off a cliff to fashion disaster. A thick waist-cinching belt is a hot accessory, but you know that it will only accentuate a tummy. So customize the trend for you: Choose narrower belts that add definition but won't make your tummy bulge more than necessary.

LEARN FROM DESIGN MASTERS OF FIT AND DISGUISE.
Michael Kors, Donna Karan, and Oscar de la Renta are all geniuses when it comes to hiding a tummy and creating the illusion of slimness. Study their collections on fashion Web sites, such as style .com, for styling tips. Print out photos, and take them shopping with you for inspiration.

BUY BIKE SHORTS IN LIVING COLOR.
Why limit yourself to shapewear in nude, black and brown when you can wear Vellum Blue, Teal Gauze, Lipstick Pink and Lilac? Spanx's new line of super thin bike shorts, called Skinny Britches, come in fifteen fashion shades so it's not so bad if you flash your Spanx when you're getting out of a car. Because these are so sheer, there are colored thongs to wear under them, which can be mixed or matched. Nothing wrong with double-Spanxing. ●

WHY THE SUDDEN BELLY

You'd be a genetic freak if you had a six-pack at forty without working out and dieting. My doctor says that six pounds is the average weight gain of a woman going through menopause. Six pounds! That may not sound like a lot, but on a petite, it's a dress size. Dr. Pamela Peeke says that there are two distinctly different types of belly fat. Menopot fat is the result of changes in estrogen levels and it encircles the waist on top of the abdomen. Doing five hundred crunches a day won't get rid of it, but limiting your caloric intake and burning the extra fat with aerobics and weight training will. Unfortunately, Peeke says, you'll always have a little roundness that you will just have to suck up! (That's why we have shapewear.) The other kind of fat, toxic fat as she calls it, lies beneath the abdominal wall and surrounds vital organs making it potentially dangerous, putting you at risk for diabetes and heart disease. A high fat diet and low activity are responsible, but genetics can play a role here, too. How to tell what kind of fat you have? Take this test: Peeke says that if you lie on your side, the menopot fat will fall to the side but the toxic fat will stay raised and firm.

10 THINGS THAT MAKE YOU LOOK FAT WHEN YOU HAVE *Buddha Belly*

1. **Showing belly** in short tops and low-rise pants or jeans. Cross this off your list forever.

2. **Cinching the waist with a wide belt** makes your belly look rounder and puffier from the side view. Either move wide belts down to navel level where they can act as camouflage or skip them.

3. **Belts at belly central.** Cut the loops off dresses or jackets that have them so you can relocate the waist slightly higher or lower instead of at the widest, fullest part of your belly.

4. **Tucking in tops**, even with tailored suits, means adding an extra layer of fabric that's guaranteed to bunch up around the tum. A snap-crotch bodysuit like those by Wolford is the only way to make a tuck-in work, since it creates a smooth line that stays in place and allows you to wear the jacket open.

5. **Wearing long fitted tees that cover your stomach isn't the answer.** Light fabrics and a taut fit only emphasize the bulge. You need to wear a loose top layer over long tees for adequate camouflage, or switch to relaxed-fit tops with strategic draping.

6. **Bathrobe-style coats and knits.** Those long cabled sweaters that look so cozy belted over turtles in catalogs make you look doughy and dumpy. Ditto, thick wool wrap overcoats.

7. **High-waist skirts and pants.** These breeze in and out of fashion, but they are worth noting because they're back now. They leave the tummy totally exposed and visible because you don't layer over a high waist. What would be the point?

8. **Heavy-duty layering.** Too many fabrics and colors stacked one on top of another like pancakes will just add pounds across your middle. Keep layers light and fluid, skimming over the body.

9. **Tight sequined tops and dresses.** So tempting, but so packed with fashion calories, and the shine factor doesn't help.

10. **Wearing waist-high** rather than high-waist pantyhose, tights, shapers, briefs.

A TUMMY-FRIENDLY GUIDE TO JACKETS

Don't you just love jackets? No other piece provides that kind of security like an extra layer of fabric buttoned up to cover your belly. They polish-up a work look or date look and free you to move and sit without worrying about your tummy or fiddling with your clothes. But, of course, there are good jackets and bad jackets when it comes to disguising the Buddha belly.

Get rid of those oversized, big-shouldered, manly looking jackets you've been hanging onto since the '80s. They not only date you, but give you a baggy, bulky shape. Even if they make a comeback, they will never make you look Fit Not Fat, so who needs them? Not you. Rather than buy a whole new wardrobe, sometimes just eliminating the bad choices in your existing wardrobe is all you need to do not to look fat! That's easy.

The jacket category has exploded with variations on classics and lots of feminine styles with collar and sleeve details that help divert the eye from the tummy. If you love the traditional navy or black blazer, it has morphed into more contemporary styles—from long and tailored boyfriend jackets to preppy shrunken crested blazers cropped at the top of the hip, which fit so close to the body that they can almost be worn without anything underneath. J. Crew, Theory, and Isaac Mizrahi for Liz Claiborne usually offer cute jackets in a range of fabrics and colors. Others, such as those by Nanette Lepore, Diane von Furstenberg, and Marc by Marc Jacobs, usually have a subtle retro feel, featuring flared peplums or A-shapes with fashion-y details such as bigger buttons and piping.

If you're job hunting and considering a new skirt or pantsuit, it's more modern now to buy a "wow" jacket separately and pair it with a sheath dress or a classic skirt. If only a traditional suit will do, make sure the jacket is a piece that you can wear over dresses, jeans, pants, and skirts already in your closet. The current crop of jackets in-store:

A-shape jacket
Fitted at shoulders and bosom then flared to an A

Blazer
Classic notch–collar lapels, single- or double-breasted

Bomber
Sporty blouson with front zip, knit bands at wrist and hem

Boyfriend blazer
Slim, elongated version to top of thigh

Cadet jacket
Military-inspired fitted jacket with stand-up collar

Cropped trench
An abbreviated trench coat cut to jacket length

Evening jacket
A dressy metallic, brocade, silk or satin

Jacket-vest
Sleeveless tailored blazer

Ladylike jacket
Straight square collarless jacket falling to the hip or just above, often seen in couture collections, in pastel tweeds and boucles

Motocross jacket
Fitted leather jacket with zip front, band collar

Pea jacket
Ladylike adaptation of the double-breasted sailor coat

Peplum jacket
Fitted to the waist with a flare to the hip

Safari jacket
Belted, patch-pocketed, with epaulettes

Short-sleeve jacket
Fitted, tailored with above-the-elbow sleeves

Shrunken blazer
Top of hip, closer-to-the-body fit

Sweater jacket
Thick, double-knit jacket/cardigan often with piping in single- or double-breasted styles

Vintage-look jacket
Cropped with three-fourth sleeves, feminine details

Unconstructed jacket
No lining, just a relaxed, tailored shape

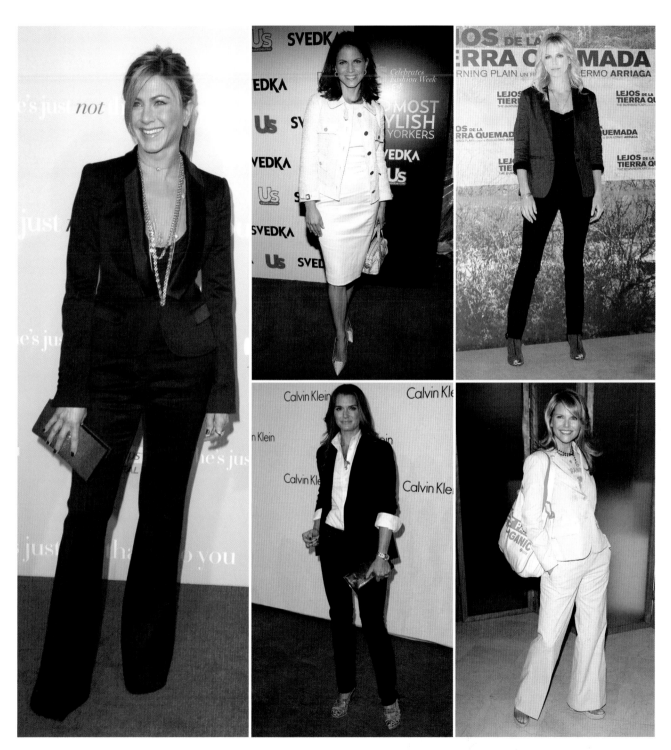

Thank you designers, for making jackets. With this kind of camouflage, who knows what lies beneath?
Clockwise from left: JENNIFER ANISTON, NATALIE MORALES, CHARLIZE THERON, CHRISTIE BRINKLEY, BROOKE SHIELDS

HIGH FAT *vs.* NO FAT

→ If you're trying to disguise a belly, you'll be most successful with a well-constructed dress designed to compress you in all the right places in a better, more forgiving fabric.

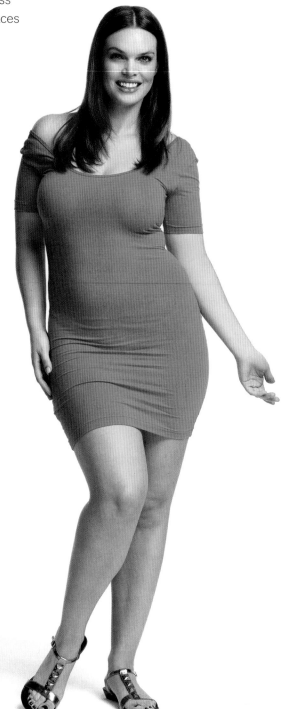

....
HIGH FAT:
The thin fabric of this stretchy T-shirt dress cradles every curve, outlining the belly and pulling across the body. The short length exposes fleshy thigh, too.

HOW FAST CAN YOU GIVE THESE AWAY?

HIGH FAT

× Belted coats in thick, stiff fabrics

× Bolero and other above-the-waist jackets

× Elastic or drawstring-waist pants, skirts

× Tight light-colored dresses

× Tucked-in tops

× Unstitched box-pleat or knife-pleat skirts

NO FAT:
This sleek yet sturdier
fabric skims past the
tummy without clinging.
The slim belt above the
actual waistline does
a good job of middle
management.

YOU CAN'T HAVE TOO MANY OF THESE!

NO FAT

√ Black A-line or sheath dresses

√ Empire and raised-waist dresses

√ Medium-width belts

√ Pencil skirts

√ Ruched tops

√ Tailored single-breasted jackets

Thinner by Tonight!

INSTANT GRATIFICATION

Throw a jacket over dark jeans. No matter what you're wearing under it, you'll have instant camouflage and feel more confident. A contemporary blazer looks slim over tanks and camisoles with dark-wash jeans.

Slip a bright jacket over a dark sheath dress. You're adding drama to a background of slimness.

Wear a high-waist body shaper with extra-firm tummy control. You can look flatter and firmer under everything from sleeveless shifts to pencil skirts.

Add a long, loose tank under your sweater as a layering piece to cover any gaps between jeans and tops.

Move your waist up or down, experiment with belts to find your best (thinnest) waistline. Try it! Take some photos—you'll be amazed.

Get immediate camouflage with draping, crossover details, tiers, or shirring that provide extra coverage without the need to layer at all. Ella Moss, Velvet, C & C California, and James Perse have the best tops.

Keep the top small and bottom voluminous . . . or keep the top voluminous and the bottom small. Fool the eye with a full drapey top and lean skirt or slimming jeans. Or, wear a fitted top with a drop-waist full skirt or wide, slouchy pants. Just choose one lane and stay in it.

Wear a dress with a deep-V neckline and a raised waist that skims past the problem. Lisa Perry comes out with this dress in hot fashion colors every season.

Go up a pant size so your flat-fronts or jeans sit slightly lower on the waist. This goes for cropped pants, too.

Slide a loose, skinny belt over a long, thin sweater to drop the attention below the waist. Slide a belt under an open cardigan or jacket for subtle waist definition. Keep the belt low on the waist, a notch looser.

Get a terrific LBD (little black dress) and wear an amazing necklace or . . .

Buy a straight or A-shaped dress with an embellished neckline. The ultimate diversionary wardrobe piece, you draw all attention away from your middle and up to your face. You need nothing more.

Hold your bag in front of your stomach, a tried-and-true celebrity trick. A big clutch works. Small dogs and babies do, too. Look for this trick in the celebrity weeklies!

BUDDHA BELLY SOLUTIONS

IF YOU'RE PETITE…

• **WEAR A FITTED BLACK DRESS** with a fancy open cardigan to bring all the attention above the waist and toward the outer silhouette. Think sequins, beads, embroidery on the cardi.

• **LOOK FOR COLOR-BLOCKED DRESSES** with strategically placed dark panels below the bosom or down the front of the dress to optically whittle your middle. Think Michelle Obama's election-night dress.

• **SHOW YOUR ARMS AND LEGS AS MUCH AS POSSIBLE** in sleeveless dresses to avoid looking too apple-y in shape. The contrast of thinner arms and legs will help deflate a tummy. If your arms really aren't that bad, get over not showing them. Really.

• **WEAR A HIP-LENGTH TUNIC OVER A SLIM SHORT SKIRT,** a great winter uniform with heeled boots; heeled sandals in summer.

IF YOU'RE SIZE 14 & UP…

• **WEAR STRAIGHT-LEG JEANS,** not skinny jeans, tapered jeans or leggings, with your blousy loose tops to avoid the dreaded ice cream cone shape.

• **LOOK FOR DRESSES THAT HAVE STRUCTURE**—A-lines and straight shifts offer controlled volume and a crisp shape.

• **TONE JACKETS AND TOPS TO MATCH OVER A CONTRASTING BASE.** Such as a camel jacket and V-neck over chocolate flat-front pants.

• **LOOK FOR JACKETS CUT TO CONTOUR AND FLOW.** Such as unconstructed jackets without linings, raglan sleeve jackets, or dolman jackets with deeper armholes instead of styles with a straight shoulder line.

• **JUST SAY NO** to the bathrobe-style winter coat.

Going to Extremes: *Middle Management*

LIPO. Lipo is a popular way to suck the fat out of a tummy, but as with any surgery, it is not without risk. Are three or four pounds of fat worth it? Up to you. But even Dr. Peeke isn't opposed to "finishing up with lipo" for women who have been exercising and eating right and still are left with a belly. Don't think that lipo is the magic bullet of weight loss, because a safe lipo, says Dr. Peeke, only removes three to four pounds of fat. She suggests that you time it right and wait till you're done losing weight through good nutrition and regular physical activity. "Don't refuse to workout and think lipo will jump start weight loss," she says. "If you drop five pounds with lipo and still have fifteen leftover to work on, that's not optimal. What do you think your stomach will look like when you're done losing? Or within five pounds of your goal?"

If you are considering lipo, do your research first. On the Web site surgery.org, sponsored by the American

BRILLIANT BUYS

BEST SHAPERS

Assets Open Bust Cami, $26; Target, target.com. Allows you to wear any style neckline. Wear your own bra.

TC Fine Intimates Strapless Bra Slip, style 4555, $66; Bloomingdale's, tcfineintimates.com. It offers double coverage with a compression panty under the slip.

Flexees Fat Free Dressing Firm Control Tank Top, style 2866, $38; Macy's, macys.com. A tummy-toning tank.

L'eggs Profiles Waist Smoother, mid-thigh, firm control, style 93444; $8.99, Wal-Mart, cvs.com. Can't beat the price of this high-waist bike short.

Wacoal Get In Shape Moderate Control Hi-Waist Long Leg Shaper, style 808123, $68; Nordstrom, barenecessities.com.

Lipo in a Box High-Waist Brief with Legs, style 46822 (open gusset), $42; lipoinabox.com or qvc.com.

Spanx Slim Cognito Shape-Suit with removable underwire, style 345, $98; spanx.com.

Spanx Hide & Sleek Slip-Suit style 114, $84; Bloomingdale's, spanx.com.

Society for Aesthetic Plastic Surgery, they issue advice, news, and warnings. Just know that there is a lot of hype out there, especially on Web sites offering the latest, greatest breakthrough treatment. The medical companies know what patients want to hear—"minimal trauma, no downtime, easy breezy." Once a doctor has invested hundreds of thousands of dollars into this new technology, don't you think that he's going to try to sell you on it the best he can? Currently, there are three kinds of lipo technologies available in the United States. Water-assisted lipo uses Jacuzzi-like nozzles. "I don't see any advantage to the water," says New York plastic surgeon Michael Kane. SmartLipo has been well marketed. Who wouldn't prefer a laser magic wand to just melt the fat away? Tumescent lipo, which is the standard lipo, is the gold standard according to Dr. Kane and other well-respected doctors, although he has high hopes for LipoSonix, which has not been approved for the United States at press time. (For more on it, see page 126).

TUMMY TUCKS. Lipo gets rid of fat cells but doesn't tighten droopy skin. With gastric bypass surgery or good old-fashioned dieting, if you drop a massive amount of weight, your whole body sags with excess skin. Dr. Peeke says, "If you've worked so hard to get rid of excess weight, why should you have to live with loose, drapey skin if you have the money for plastic surgery?" A tummy tuck (abdominoplasty) might be the solution. After their final pregnancy, some women choose to have the tummy tuck done right after delivery, with a plastic surgeon, of course. One caveat: Dr. Pamela Peeke says women who have had successive C-sections, or more than one pregnancy and at least one C-section, can have same belly-jelly issues even after a tummy tuck. Another reason to own shapewear. Downside: This is major surgery and may require three days in the hospital. ●

Vows *for* Buddha Belly

☐ **I WILL** learn to love shapewear bike shorts.

☐ **I WILL** buy a dress instead of a skirt or pants next time I need something to wear for a special occasion.

☐ **I WILL** get over the number and go up a size if it looks better.

☐ **I WILL** replace my short tees and tanks with longer versions.

☐ **I WILL NOT** blame my belly on my pregnancy now that my kid is ten.

☐ **I WILL** lighten up on myself, knowing that every woman gains an average of six pounds with menopause. Big deal.

DON'T YOU DARE...

Cinch a four-inch belt around your waist in a tight knit. Your belly will look like it's popping out under it.

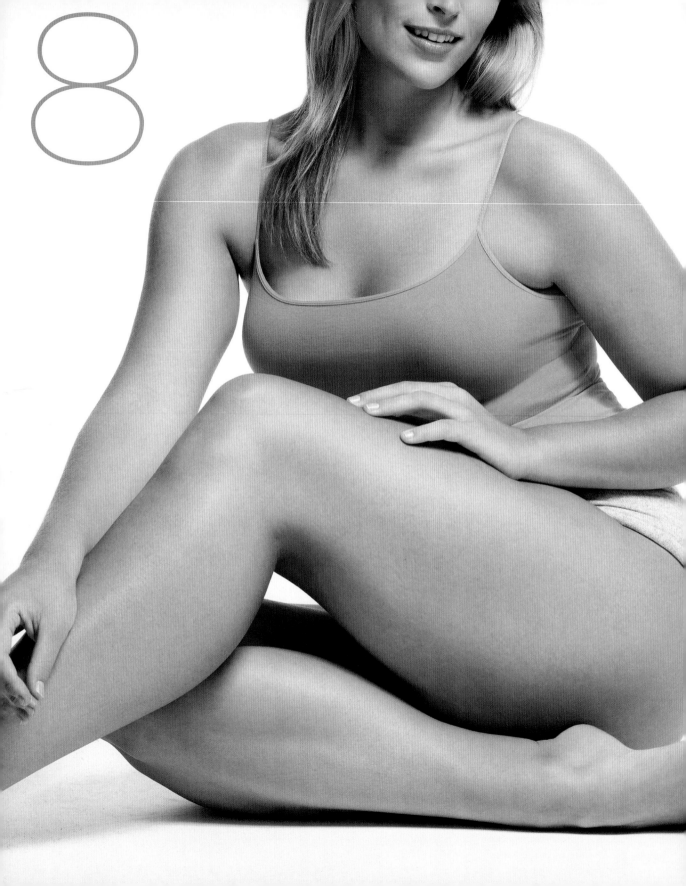

8

Wide Hips + Thighs

AKA
Thunder thighs,
drumstick legs,
kissing thighs,
saddlebags,
ham hocks,
birthing hips,
bottom heavy,
poulkes,
lightbulb legs

YOU KNOW YOU HAVE IT WHEN...

Oh, let's face it, this one you just know you have . . . Your thighs rub together when you walk . . . There's no space between your thighs when your knees are together . . . Pants always look like they're pulling around the crotch . . . You're a hula hoop champ . . . You're thinking of taking up Hawaiian dancing.

→ Raise your hand if "pear shape" is the silhouette that best describes your hips and thighs. I hear you—and my hand is up there, too. While Beyoncé is working overtime trying to bring hourglass-shaped sexy back, it's not back yet; and those of us who have ample hips and thighs know too well that Marilyn Monroe's kind of va-va-va-voom is not such a glamorous asset when you're trying on dresses, skirts, and pants today. If you have hips, you have hips, and there is not that much you can do about your actual bone structure. So let's stop denigrating our bodies and blaming ourselves. Only you can answer this question: Is it my fat that's making me look fat or is it my clothes that are making me look fat? On me, it's a little of both. So, until that day comes when I reach my ideal body weight, I'm going to follow the advice in this chapter and stop buying all those fattening clothes that only give a shout-out to my hips and thighs. Like that beaded and sequin snakeskin Dolce & Gabbana skirt—what was I thinking?!

YOUR DRESS-THINNER STRATEGY
for Wide Hips + Thighs

You've heard the expression, there's more than one way to get downtown?
Well, to get Fit Not Fat hips and thighs, you have your choice of several routes.

ROUTE #1
BALANCE BOULEVARD

If you're a classic pear shape, your hips and thighs are larger than your shoulders and your bust. So, your mission is to create a sense of balance between your upper and lower halves. You can accomplish this in one of two ways: *1)* By increasing the width of your upper half so it's as wide as your bottom half or *2)* by compressing your lower half so it's as trim as your top half. The way to go really depends on your size. If you're tiny on top, go ahead and bulk up your shoulders and bust with shoulder pads, a padded bra, or shoulder accoutrements, like epaulettes—you need it. If you're already big on top, don't throw on a moo-moo and call it a day—it will just make you look big and shapeless all over. You do want to shrink your bottom half, as you want to look smaller overall and minimize the hips/thighs. The fastest way to take inches off is to trade up from panties as usual to shapewear bike shorts under skirts and dresses, and a capri-length shaper under pants and jeans.

ROUTE #2
DISAPPEARANCE DRIVE

If you want to make your heavy bottom half disappear from sight, you don't have to be David Copperfield, but you do need to create a waist-up world for yourself, one in which you give others absolutely no reason to look at you below the belt. How? By keeping your bottom half unimportant. That means no boy shorts, shorts of any kind, hot pants, micro-minis, poufs, ruffles, tiers, loud prints, floral prints, animal prints, cargo pants, white pants, harem pants, leather pants, crushed velvet

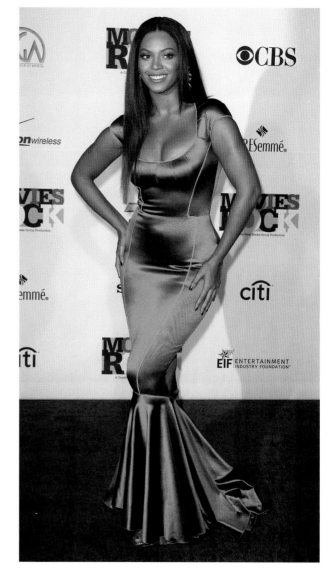

This girl is working overtime to bring hourglass-shaped sexy back! It can't happen soon enough. Go, BEYONCÉ!

pants, fancy pants, screaming neon colors, or balloon hemlines. Save the party for your top half—that's where you will seduce, dazzle, and entertain the latest trends.

ROUTE #3
REDIRECTION ROAD

As you get dressed each morning, remember that you are in control of where you want others to focus. You need to redirect everyone's attention from the extra poundage down there, but to where? To your body part that is most delicate, feminine, and bony. Don't say you don't have one! If you have great shoulders, how about an off-the-shoulder sweater, one-shoulder dress, or a halter top? If you have good arms and a nice neckline, collarbone, and décolletage, wear strapless tops, V-necks, scoop necks, and boat necks. If you have a great bust, long-chain necklaces, gorgeous beads, charms on a cord, or vintage-inspired medallions will do the trick. If you have small waist, cinch it! Wear a belt over pants, jeans, skirts, dresses, and cardigans. If you're petite, stick to delicate, ladylike one- or two-inch belts. Big, chunky belts dripping with chains require a long enough torso to handle three to five inches of leather. You can also cinch your waist with a form-fitting jacket, blazer, or top. And if you're thinnest right under your bra band, go for a trendy empire-waist dress or top (no pregnancy required). ●

10 THINGS THAT MAKE YOU LOOK FAT WHEN YOU HAVE
Wide Hips + Thighs

1. **Skinny jeans tucked into boots**

2. **Tight boot-leg jeans**

3. **Wrap sweaters or sarongs tied around the hips**

4. **Boyfriend sweaters with big bulky pockets**

5. **Tops that gather at the widest part of your thighs**

6. **Whiskers across the crotch on pants, skirts**

7. **Jackets, sweaters, vests that hit mid-thigh**

8. **Cargo pockets on the thigh**

9. **A peasant skirt that tiers across the hips**

10. **Micro-minis and shorts**

JEANS AND PANTS THAT WILL FLATTER YOUR
HIPS + THIGHS

Wide-leg and straight-leg jeans and trousers are best for skimming thighs and hips. Conversely, anything that hugs and tapers at the ankles will turn your legs into two chicken drumsticks. Pants that are too tight on the upper leg will make your thighs look like sausages desperately trying to break free from their casing, so stay away from boot-cut jeans, liquid jeans or second-skin leathers—not a good look!

Look for flat-front pants with wide legs and a natural waistline. Your best pants will fall straight down from the waist so there are no lumps, bumps, or bulges sticking out at the thigh. So sell all your old clothes at a yard sale and plan to spend some of the profits on a new pair of pants! Here's your shopping checklist:

LOOK FOR A MEDIUM RISE. It will lengthen the torso and minimize full hips and thighs. They should fit easily and comfortably over the hips.

DON'T BUY THEM IF THEY ARE BUNCHING, CREASING, OR PULLING AROUND THE CROTCH AND FLY—a major fashion faux pas. Sit down on a chair in the dressing room or in the store to make sure they don't crinkle up right there.

PASS OVER ANY PAIR WITH PLEATS AS IF THEY WERE POISONOUS...BECAUSE THEY ARE! All you need is one precise, razor-sharp crease down the front and back of your pants to elongate and slim your thighs. If the pants don't have a crease, iron one in or get them pressed at the dry cleaner. (But not on jeans, please.)

NO POCKETS! If you fall in love with pants that have bulky side pockets, you can have your tailor remove the pocket bags and sew them closed. Some angled side pockets can be flattering but no pockets are better.

SWAP-OUTS:
WAYS TO HIDE THE EVIDENCE

Instead of	→	Go for
An animal print skirt		An animal print top
A boyfriend blazer		Cropped, curvy jacket
Flats		Heels
A mid-thigh cardi		Short cardi
A scarf as a belt		A belt as a belt
Short shorts		Knee-length skirts
Tapered pants		Wide-leg pants
A printed peasant skirt		A straight skirt in a dark solid

YOUR HIPS-AND-THIGH-FRIENDLY GUIDE TO SKIRTS

What you don't want from now on are compliments on your skirt. They don't mean that your skirt is flattering, but rather that your hips/thighs are not going unnoticed. Let's go to the closet. See any skirts that have ruching, beading, pleating, tiers, ruffles, lace, or eyelet? How about anything black leather, hot pink silk, tie-dyed, sequined, tulle, or glittery? Stuff them into a shopping bag and call the nearest charity for pickup. Sorry, but you want to look thinner, don't you?

Now let's look at the volume of the rest of your skirts. Fuller skirts like peasant skirts and dirndls may make you feel comfortable because they are more forgiving, but let's be real; you can hide a small animal under there and no one would be the wiser! They are loaded with calories. A full skirt can make you look fuller and a pouf skirt can make you look, well, pouffy. We don't need any more volume; we're trying to play down the lower half.

Don't even think about miniskirts or skirts and dresses with a high slit; you don't want to offer the world a peep show of your kissing thighs. As for hemlines, don't go more than two inches above the knee or you'll be entering a flab zone. At-the-knee hemlines may be your most flattering.

Be wary of the A-line skirt. It may seem like a logical, safe choice, but if it is a severe A-line,

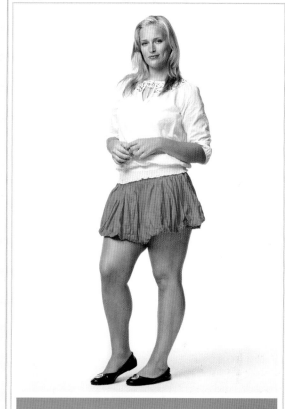

DON'T GO THERE

Only ballerinas and four-year-olds can look slim in a skirt this fattening. Yummy, but too many calories.

it will create a triangle effect from your hips to your knees. The A-line not only adds girth, it can also look dowdy. If you have any A-lines that need to become straight skirts, bring them to your tailor for this simple alteration. Straight skirts will give you a sexy shape, so will pencil skirts if they're not too tight. Fit and flare skirts as well as trumpet and tulip-shaped skirts in fabrics with a Lycra® blend will also contain and shape your thighs. Make sure to wear compression shapewear underneath these shapely skirts to suck it all in!

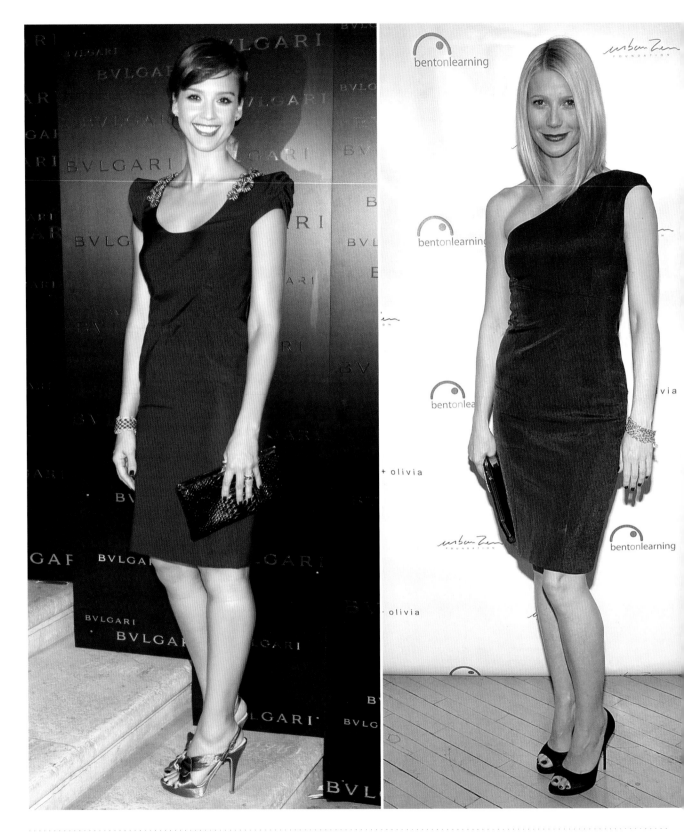

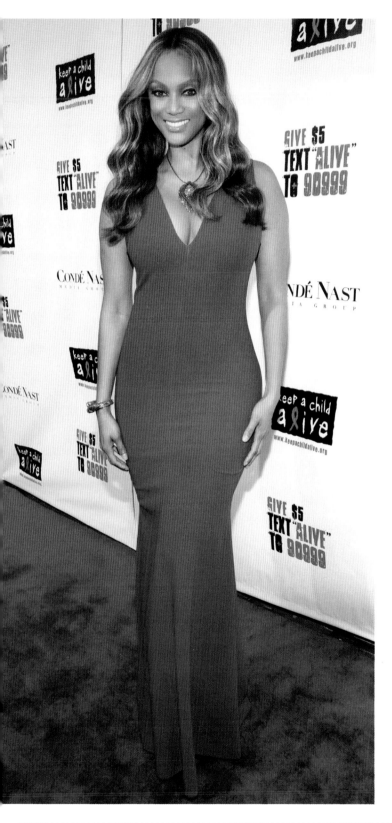

These women have no problem admitting that they wear Spanx; in fact, some even admit to double-Spanxing!
JESSICA ALBA
GWYNETH PALTROW
TYRA BANKS

Bye-Bye, Briefs!

Time to say good-bye to underwear as we know it. See ya later, thongs! *Hasta la vista*, bikinis! Most panties hit in all the wrong places if you have generous hips and thighs. Who needs that bulge where the elastic meets the flesh? "I wear Spanx every single day. I've given up panties," Oprah revealed on her show a few seasons ago. If you want to look Fit Not Fat daily, why not join those who just say no to unsupportive undies? The bigger (and older) we get, the more help we need from our underwear, so compression shapewear, here we come! I must have twenty or so pairs of shapewear bike shorts in my lingerie drawer, from various brands offering different degrees of compression. Some days you need to be slurped in to the max; others you don't. Look for bike shorts that will not create a line across your thighs to wear with skirts and dresses. When you're wearing jeans or pants, you want the capri-length shapers that end at the knees or ankles. For the best shapers out now, see Brilliant Buys, page 126.

HIGH FAT *vs.* NO FAT

→ Stop shopping for trendy skirts. It's smarter to indulge your upper half in fattening frills, such as ruffles, bows, poufs, eyelet and the color white. Instead, scour the racks for the perfect black skirt that shaves off inches without screaming "Look at me. Look at me!"

HIGH FAT:
Could this skirt hit at a worse spot? Aside from being too short, it attracts the eye with fading, loose-hanging threads and horizontal lines at the hem.

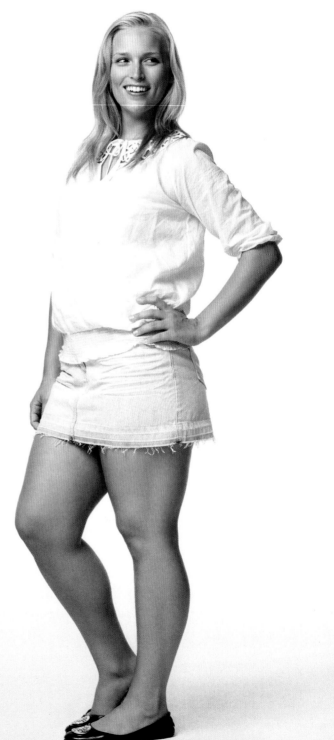

HOW FAST CAN YOU GIVE THESE AWAY?

HIGH FAT

× Cargo pants

× Leggings as pants

× Micro-minis and shorts

× Pleated pants and skirts

× Pouffy skirts

What a difference!

The micro-mini can't compete with a knee-grazer when you want your thighs to look de-sized.

NO FAT:
This shapely pencil skirt fashions the body into a sexy hourglass. Black opaque tights and high heel pumps create a long, continuous line from hips to toes.

YOU CAN'T HAVE TOO MANY OF THESE!

NO FAT

√ Dark denim jeans

√ Fifties-style cocktail dresses

√ Roomy knee-length pencil skirts

√ Wide-leg pants

√ Wrap dresses

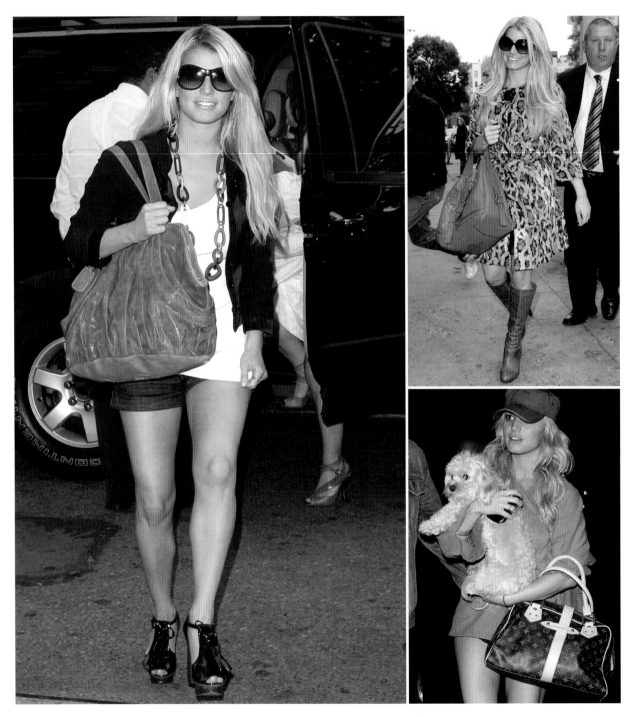

Objects strategically placed in front of the middle is a paparazzi favorite.
JESSICA SIMPSON is a skilled practitioner.

HIDING FAT WITH YOUR BAG

Don't want to lose weight? Carry an eye-catching tote, and hide your rolls on the side. "If your bag is an interesting conversation piece, people are looking at the bag instead of how much weight you've gained," says Kim Isaacsohn, who knows about hiding fat with bags, as head coachman of the Clever Carriage Handbag Company. To make this trick work, the size of your bag has to be in proportion to your size. "Big girl, small clutch and it looks like you're carrying a lunchbox. Small girl, big bag, you look like you should be inside the bag." Kim applies her same theory for blocking bulge to dogs. "If you're a big girl, you look fatter carrying a small dog; you need medium-size dog." Got it.

DON'T WASTE A PENNY ON . . .

ANTI-CELLULITE TREATMENTS

In the fight against cellulite, women are too willing to try anything. Why waste money on treatments and products that offer such fleeting results?

ENDERMOLOGIE is a massage machine with rollers and a suction action. If you've ever had it done, it feels like a vacuum cleaner is sucking up your skin . . . it's painful. "These machines beat up the skin, which causes a little swelling, making the skin look smoother for a little while," says New York plastic surgeon Michael Kane. "You're damaging the superficial fat a bit, but then it just goes back to normal." That's a lot of pain for not a lot of gain.

CELLULITE CREAMS, if they worked, they would have removed the dimpled lumps on Kate Moss, Nicole Kidman, Eva Longoria Parker, Paris Hilton, and all the other celebrities who show up in the weeklies with cottage cheese thighs.

Every time I sit front row at a fashion show, I'm kind of relieved to see that stick-thin, drop-dead-gorgeous models on the catwalk have cellulite, too. Nothing topical gets rid of cellulite completely. Yes, some creams may make your cellulite less apparent temporarily—i.e., for a few hours—but nobody can prove that the creams can penetrate the skin deeply enough to reach fat cells. If you're heading to the beach and need a quick fix, a body cream with caffeine will temporarily smooth skin by reducing water retention, but we're talking a few hours at best.

ANTI-CELLULITE STOCKINGS, again, fall into the category of, we wish! We wish we could just put on a pair of stockings and banish cellulite forever. The fine print on one package says that you need to wear these stockings five days a week for a minimum of eight weeks before any results can be seen, and even then they promise only to reduce the appearance of cellulite, not eliminate it. That's a huge commitment for not a lot of reward.

NEWSFLASH! Dr. Michael Kane and other doctors are optimistic about a new machine called LipoSonix, which painlessly delivers high-frequency focused ultrasound to the superficial fat and kills the fat cells. "Once you kill the fat cells, the body digests them and doesn't produce them anymore—they're gone forever," he explains. "It's like a nonsurgical, noninvasive liposuction." At press time, it was still in clinical trial and had not yet gone for FDA approval, though it's currently available in Canada and Europe. If it really does work, you'll know about it . . . there will be lines around the block!

WHAT ELSE YOU CAN DO

Spinning. While it won't get rid of cellulite (I spin and still have it), it will take inches off your hips and thighs. I see the difference on myself and on the narrow "boy bodies" that populate my spin class. "Spinning is one of the most efficient fat burners for your hips and thighs," says Ruth Zukerman, co-founder of the spin studio, Soul-Cycle, in New York City. "If there's a more efficient way to burn fat in forty-five minutes, I haven't found it. You work every muscle in your legs up to your gluts. But it's not about spot reducing. Spinning is cardio work so you lose fat everywhere."

BRILLIANT BUYS

SHAPEWEAR

L'eggs Profiles Capri, style 93434, $8.99; Wal-Mart, cvs.com. Thigh control at a nice price. Runs small.

TC Fine Intimates Just Enough High-Waist Bike Pant with Wonderful Edge, style 4019, $38; barenecessities.com or for stores, see cupidintimates.com.

Wacoal Get In Shape Moderate Control Long Leg Brief 805123, $55; Nordstrom, bareneccessites.com.

Spanx Slim Cognito Shaping Mid-Thigh Bodysuit, style 067, $72; Bloomingdale's, spanx .com.

Spanx Hide & Sleek Half Slip, style 054A, $52; Bloomingdale's, spanx.com.

Donna Karan The Body Perfect Collection, Waist Embrace Capri (Style #A919). It comes a little below the bust line and is Capri Length. It is retailing for $55.00 at saks.com.

Vows *for* Wide Hips + Thighs

- ☐ **I WILL** always wear dark on my bottom half.

- ☐ **I WILL** choose straight-leg jeans or wide-leg jeans over the boot-cut, which can hug a thick thigh.

- ☐ **I WILL** stay away from pleats and side pockets because they add extra calories.

- ☐ **I WILL** steer clear of drawstring and cargo pants.

- ☐ **I WILL NEVER** wear tapered pants.

- ☐ **I WILL NOT** wear tops that stop where my hips are fullest.

- ☐ **I WILL NOT** wear hip-hugging anything!

DON'T YOU DARE...

Wear a shirtdress that buttons all the way down your body; that dreaded pull on the buttons around your hips will keep eyes focused on all the wrong places. Instead, go for a wrap dress that will draw attention to your waist and the upper half of your body.

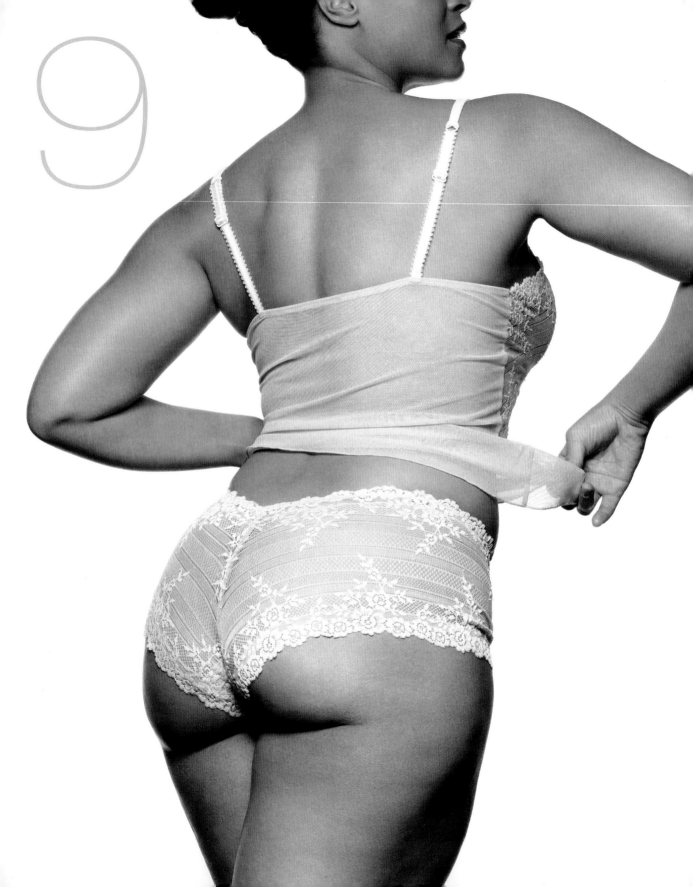

Big Booty

bootylicious,
tuchus, junk
in the trunk,
bubble butt,
wide load,
bodonkadonk,
baby got back,
buns, keister,
rump

YOU KNOW YOU HAVE IT WHEN...

Pants are tight on the butt, roomy at the waist . . . You can hold a pencil underneath your butt cheek . . . You think that movie theater seats are a bit small . . . People can identify you from your backside . . . Pants have been known to rip at the seams . . . You feel like your butt leaves the room five minutes after you do.

→ Booties are having their moment. Ever since Jennifer Lopez and Beyoncé brought bootylicious into the lexicon, women with prominent posteriors no longer feel they must cover their butts. If you're at peace with your assets and want to celebrate this body part, don't let anyone stop you. Just do the opposite of all the advice in this chapter!

For those who prefer the no-butt look and are trying to downsize their derrieres, you've no doubt uttered these words at least once in your lifetime: "Does my butt look fat in this?" and thought it a zillion times. There's a reason why, when we try something on, the first thing most of us do is spin around to check out our backside. When your rear end looks good, you look good. And, on the flip side, when your gluteus maximus looks too pronounced, it kills your overall look. How to disguise an obvious behind? You need a strategy, because what we forget is that just as many people see us going as coming—so cramming yourself into a pair of too-tight jeans doesn't work!

YOUR DRESS-THINNER STRATEGY
for a Big Booty

→ THE STRATEGY HERE IS A TWO-parter: First, you want to get your tush under control in the best shape possible, and then you want to do everything you can to hide it from view. Why would you do that? The smaller you can get it, the easier it will be for you and everyone else to forget about it.

PART ONE: RESCULPT

Smaller! Rounder! Higher! It's amazing what you can do with shapewear these days to resculpt your bottom and position it where you want it. While some women lament about a big bum, others complain of a flat fanny, saggy haunches, or butt cleavage. Fake out your particular issues with shapewear, but beware of the "bubble butt" or "uni-butt"—that shape you get from an old-fashioned girdle, which resembles a big, round ball without any cheek definition. "The uni-butt look is a dead giveaway that you're wearing shapewear," says Spanx's Misty Elliott. "It flattens your backside for a not-so natural look." No reason for that when you can choose from state-of-the-art brands that have "zoned" compression. Your perfect shaper can do a lot:

1) Take inches off your backside

2) Give your butt a lift

3) Get rid of butt cleavage

4) Stop the jiggling

5) Cover dimpling

6) Separate your cheeks

7) Make you look better than you do naked. If you're not a shapewear devotee right now, don't worry, you'll be one by the end of this book (for Brilliant Buys, see page 140).

PART TWO: COVER YOUR BUTT

The right clothes are those that are loose enough to easily flow over your entire backside so that everything's covered, nothing's showing, and your butt is a nonissue. The best you can hope for? That no one takes notice of your behind. Curate a closet full of jackets, coats, coatdresses, sweaters, tunics, and cardigans that cover your butt. If you are petite, avoid mid-thigh length cover-ups and split the difference with hip-grazing jackets, cardis, and tops. Your Fit Not Fat tip: Make sure these covering pieces are structured enough to nip in at the waist and give you an hourglass shape. New York City fashion coach Susan Sommers of Dresszing, tells clients, "Better if your cover-ups are a thin layer. Fabric that is too bulky or heavy will add volume. You don't

want to look like solid mass from your shoulders on down." Belts are big now, but watch the size, she warns. "Cinching your waist with a thick belt will make your butt look bigger."

When people stare at your rump, it generally means that something is off. Too-tight clothes, like pants that cut up between your butt cheeks or pencil skirts or shift dresses that outline your rear end, only accentuate an ample behind. You don't want anything clinging to your rear, ever. So choose a straight-cut or wide-leg trouser, and the pant will fall straight from your hips. You don't want any kind of pants that narrow at the bottom, such as tapered, capris, or harem. You want flat-front pants in weighty fabrics that fall gently over your curves. No cuffs, side pockets on the seam, or pleats—we don't need the extra baggage.

Because you want to redirect the eyes of the world anywhere but your butt, you want to silence all rear-end hubbub. Keep it quiet back there by rejecting loud details such as contrast stitching, grommets, rivets, bows, buttons, buckles, gathers, pleats, shine, rhinestones, bleaching, logos—basically anything that's not chic, simple, and subdued. In other words, you don't want to wear

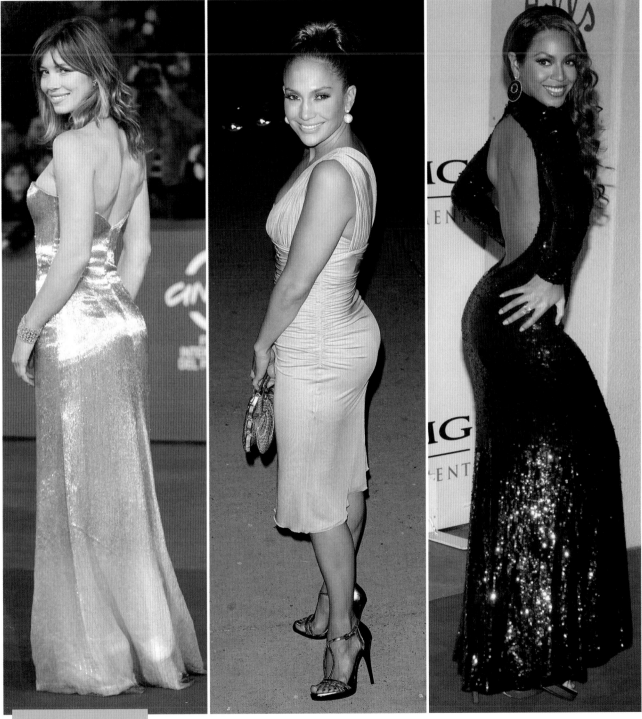

Working it

A high, rounded, toned derriere can be a bootiful thing. These stars know how to maximize their assets. JESSICA BIEL, JENNIFER LOPEZ, BEYONCÉ

A BUTT-FRIENDLY
GUIDE TO PANTS

Are you wearing elastic-waist pants right now? They're extremely comfy, but they're the worst kind of pants you can wear if you don't want to look fat. The loosely gathered fabric in the back does nothing to shape you and only adds more girth to your rear. Another reason to avoid them is that, when you slip them on day after day, you can't tell if you've gained or lost weight because they always fit (as opposed to a pair of slacks with a button and zipper). Because they are so easy to hide in, you can easily disconnect from your body. Dr. Pamela Peeke discourages women from wearing them when they come to her office. The mind-body connection is so powerful, she wants her patients to be conscious of their bodies. Big clothes that you can hide out in are not helpful when you're trying to remove excess weight—and not look fat.

I know that this is a daunting challenge, especially for those who have been buying nothing but elastic pants for years. So, wean yourself off them at your own pace. Getting rid of the elastic pants in your closet might fall into the category WIMP (When I'm Mentally Prepared). You'll do it, eventually, you just don't want to go cold turkey right now . . . believe me, I get it.

What pants to wear? Flared boot-cut or straight-leg trousers are a godsend for curvy girls because they create a straight line from butt to feet, so your bottom isn't the main focus. The higher the waistband, the more observable the butt, which is why "mom jeans" are so damning. High-waisted pants only look great on women with elongated, slender torsos. If you're short waisted—think about it—your breasts will touch the waistband and hide your torso. On the back of pants, besom pockets (which look like slits, set into the fabric) are better than patch pockets (which are sewn on and attached) because they don't add unnecessary bulk. Pants without pockets can be flattering, too, though jeans without pockets are not.

pink sweatpants that say the name of your high school, college, football team, or a logo across the rump for all to read! In this case, just repeat the mantra: Plain is good. Boring is good!

BE PICKY WHEN SHOPPING FOR JEANS

If I had to give the Most Flattering award to just a single piece of clothing in my closet, it would have to be my boot-cut dark denim jeans. Why? They miraculously give me someone else's tush—and shape and boost it as well. I know what my rear end looks like . . . and it pales in comparison to what I see in the mirror when I'm wearing these jeans! To find your dream jeans, you have to be picky.

BE PICKY ABOUT YOKES.

You probably never gave much thought to the yoke on a pair of jeans. Yokes are that horizontal strip of fabric that runs between the pockets and the waist. Yokes that form a V-shape, as opposed to a straight line, will work exactly like a V-neck top and minimize your behind. It all helps.

BE PICKY ABOUT POCKETS.

Their placement is critical when it comes to showcasing your best bottom line. Go for larger pockets that ride high on the seat and are close together, rather than those that sit low on the seat and are spaced far apart. Too low, and they'll bring your rear down with them. Too teeny, and they'll make a wide expanse of rear-end real estate look more significant in comparison. Jeans that have flaps with buttons with pockets are actually saying, "Look at my butt." One brand that has perfected the art of pocket placement is Habitual. "To give the butt a lift, all of our pockets are strategically placed beneath the yoke," says Habitual's brand director Renée Raimondi-Jaco. Stay away from pocketless jeans—pockets provide visual distraction.

BE PICKY ABOUT STYLE.

The most flattering silhouettes are boot cut and straight leg. The third choice is a wide-leg jean that works for work (in a casual office) and is a chic alternative to relaxed-fit jeans. You just have to try these styles on to see what gives you the best all-over proportion. For example, a boot cut can balance out a heavy mid-section but it is not going to flatter a thick thigh. If you are not in proportion, a straight leg might fit even better.

BE PICKY ABOUT RISE.

High-rise jeans are mom jeans—avoid at all costs. Super-low-risers will give you butt cleavage. Best is a medium-low-rise, which is a nine-inch rise from waistband to crotch. Ample butts may avoid the too-tight-in-the-crotch issue with jeans that feature a lower rise in front, higher rise in back.

BE PICKY ABOUT FABRICATION.

Don't buy jeans without stretch. Stretch gives jeans a glove-like fit without the diaper-bottom sag. You want denim with about 2 percent spandex or Lycra®. Contrary to what you may think, stretch doesn't mean tight—jeans made with spandex or Lycra® actually have give and will comfortably conform to your bottom in the most flattering way. A new generation of Lycra®, XFit Lycra®, is now in some of the hottest names in jeans, brands such as J Brands, Joe's Jeans, Serfontaine, True Religion, and AG. Its "breakthrough" patented cross-weave technology helps slenderize curves.

BE PICKY ABOUT FIT.

Jeans should fit your tush to perfection—they can easily be taken in everywhere else. Never buy jeans

SWAP-OUTS:
WAYS TO HIDE THE BUTT

Instead of	Go for
Bikini panties	Thongs or bike shorts
Cigarette pants	Straight-leg pants
Floral print pants	Floral print top
Gathered, tight layering tee	Empire-waist top
High-rise mom jean	Mid-low-rise jean
Jeans with a light wash	Dark denim jeans
Jeans with small pockets	Jeans with large back pockets
A leather pencil skirt	A leather jacket
Opaques, fishnets	Control-top opaques, fishnets
Tapered pants	Boot-cut pants

THE CASE FOR ONE
GREAT PAIR OF JEANS

If you're like most women in America, chances are your rear is swathed in denim most of the time. Jeans are such a beloved staple of most women's wardrobes because they have a much longer life span than dresses, skirts, and pants and can be worn in a range of settings and occasions, depending on your styling. That is why it's worth investing in at least one fabulous pair that you can wear with heels at night (the longer your legs, the thinner you'll look). According to *Women's Wear Daily*, jeans priced between $10 and $30 account for 53 percent of the overall denim market, with the average price of jeans coming in at $24.50. If you can find a pair of jeans that makes your butt look amazing for less than $25, go for it. That means that your booty is shapely on its own and doesn't need the extra help of a pair designed for maximum minimizing and lift. Like the model in our No Fat photo, who is wearing her own jeans from the Gap.

Did you know that women in the United States (according to a 2009 Cotton Inc. survey) own an average of seven pairs of jeans? If, out of all the jeans you own, you don't have one pair that makes you look Fit Not Fat, then I suggest you try a little experi-ment. First, do the math: Add up how much you've spent on jeans that don't do much for you. For instance, seven pairs of jeans at $25 a pair is $175. So go to your nearest department store and try on jeans priced up to $175. Take them home, try them on again, and compare them to all the jeans in your closet. Have someone take a photo of you from the back, side, and front in each pair of jeans. If the new jeans are far superior in fit, and make you so happy you never want to take them off, you might convince yourself to take a fresh approach to shopping: Buy less, buy better! Do you think that anyone will notice or care that you're wearing the same jeans you wore last week? You could have bought mul-tiple pairs of the same jean because it fit so well!

Remember, that at midlife, it's not about how much we have in our clos-ets but the way each piece makes us feel when we put it on. And, when you amortize the cost per wear of this one pair of jeans over the years, you'll owe them money!

The right pair of jeans is like a bra for your butt . . . it will shrink, minimize, shape and lift. What brands create the best bottom line? See Brilliant Buys, page 140.

you can't pull up the zipper on. They should be snug, but not too tight. They'll stretch a little bit once you wear them. Try jeans on in front of a three-way mirror to get a good view. May I repeat here? Try jeans on in front of a three-way mirror to get a great rear view. Bend down like you're picking something off the floor—if you see any butt cleav-age, toss those jeans to the side. Never buy jeans that are too small right now, but you plan on fitting in them when you lose those last ten pounds. Those jeans will sit in your closet, taunting you every time you look at them.

BE PICKY ABOUT BUTT-LIFT.

If you're saggy or flat, the right pair of jeans can rescue your rump from going downhill. "Stay away from a really high rise, because it will flat-ten you out and give you '70s mom butt,'" says Raimondi of Habitual. The rise on their Grace jean is nine inches, an inch and half higher than their standard rise, just enough to cover muffin top (see Chapter 6 for more on that) but not high enough to flatten your rear. And check out the butt-lifters from Joe's Jeans (Honey style), Paige Premium Denim (Hollywood Hills), 7 For All Mankind (High Rise Boot Cut), and J Brand (Scarlett). •

JEANS THAT MAKE YOU LOOK FAT WHEN YOU HAVE

A BIG BOOTY

The latest trends that will look amazing – on Kate Moss!

Like everything else in fashion retail, denim sales have been challenged. Because jeans last so long, we don't need to buy a new pair every season. So denim brands work their butts off to entice you with a hot new trend. Unless the trend is flattering on you, don't succumb. Stick to what works—clean, simple, dark denim, with a little stretch—and you'll look Fit Not Fat.

ACID-WASH JEANS

These '80s flashbacks didn't look good when we were two sizes smaller. Here's a general rule about the '80s: Don't go back.

BLING JEANS

Stay in Vegas. Keep your jeans clean! Stars, designs, or logos spelled in rhinestones are high fat.

BOYFRIEND JEANS

Baggy, casual, and worn-looking, they're too shapeless. Leave these where they belong— in his closet.

BRIGHT JEANS

The electric company of jeans— from orange to lime green, hot pink and Day-Glo yellow—are fattening. And in corduroy? Double the calories!

LIQUID LEGGINGS AND RESIN-COATED JEANS

These are glossy black or metallic jeans that make you look like you were poured into them. Unless you want to dress as Olivia Newton-John in *Grease* for Halloween, you don't need your butt amplified in such a tight, shiny way.

RIPPED JEANS

Hard to take a grown woman seriously with holes across her butt or thighs. Say no to holes, whiskers, abrasions, and distressing; they make you appear shorter and fatter when it's a long, lean leg you're after.

SKINNY JEANS

Skinny jeans are for skinny models. They do nothing to accommodate a real woman's curves.

A BUTT-FRIENDLY GUIDE TO SKIRTS

You need skirts that are longer than they are wide.

Think vertical rectangle as opposed to horizontal square. So that micro-mini skirt is not going to work. Everyone says that A-lines are the most flattering, but I have to tell you, A-lines can be frumpy. If you choose an A-line, make sure that it is not an exaggerated A—you don't want to look like a triangle. If you have an A-line that fits well in the butt but extends too far at the knee, take it to your tailor and have it made into a straight skirt by taking it in a few inches. A straight skirt that is not too tight in the bum is good, as long as it hovers around the knee. You can even wear a moderate pencil if it's not so tight that it outlines your tush. There are some skirts you should split with. If you're not ready yet, just put them aside at the back of your closet and see if you wear them in a year. If not, good riddance. Here's a quick Do Not Wear list (more on skirts, next chapter): ankle length, ballerina, boxy, dirndl, full, minis, micro-minis, pleated, drop waist, busy prints, peasant, and tutus.

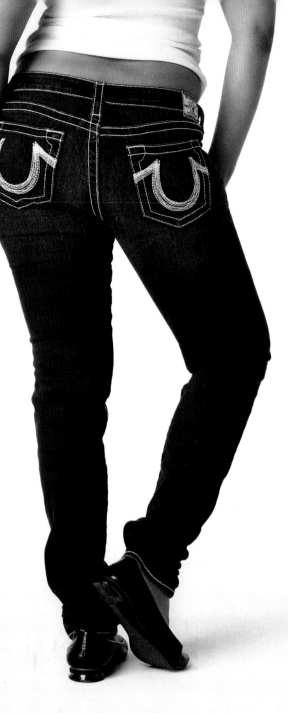

HIGH FAT:
Jeans this flashy shouldn't
even enter the dressing
room. Heed the High Fat
warning signs:
1. Bold white stitching
2. Low pockets
3. Skinny legs

HIGH FAT *vs.* NO FAT

→ The right pair of jeans is like a bra for your bum. Instead of straps and bands, you have pockets and yokes that can minimize, shape, and bring up the rear. It's all about mastering the secret language of pockets, where placement is pretty much everything.

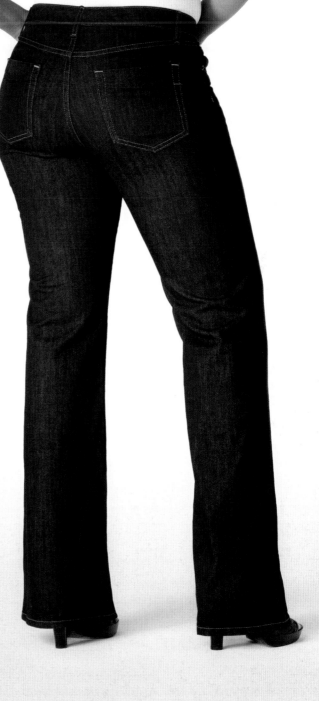

NO FAT:
Love a clean, dark denim
jean: Nothing much to
catch the eye—no logos,
tags, grommets, or decorative
extras. Higher pockets lift
you up where you belong.

What a difference!

*Butt makeover:
Why look low, wide, and
flattened out (High Fat)
when you can look higher,
smaller, and rounder
(No Fat)?*

Thinner by Tonight!

INSTANT GRATIFICATION

Keep your entire outfit monochrome.

Choose black, brown, navy, or gray over white, yellow, pink, or orange for your bottom.

Wrap solid colors, not florals or Pucci-esque prints, around your rear.

Put on the highest heels you own.

Wear footless pantyhose under a long summer dress.

Select basic, simple, and clean lines—no ruffles, poufs, cuffs, or folds.

Go for dull, flat fabrics—nothing shiny, slippery, sheer, or metallic.

Pull on a pair of dark jeans and high-heeled boots.

Toss on a tunic that reaches the bottom of your behind.

Step into a pair of black opaque tights with compression.

Lose visible panty lines with a thong, G-string, or cheeky.

Slide into a bike short that lifts and separates your booty.

Close the gap at the waist with a belt or a button.

Throw on a bright, cheery, three-quarter trench coat.

Zip into a solid-colored A-line dress.

BIG BOOTY SOLUTIONS

IF YOU'RE PETITE...

• DO HAVE A LOOK IN THE PETITE DEPARTMENT. Petite jeans are so in demand that in some stores, they are the first to go.

• BEWARE OF HIGH WAISTED WIDE-LEG PANT. You might drown in it.

IF YOU'RE SIZE 14 & UP...

• MOST BRANDS ONLY GO TO UP TO 32 IN JEANS. "Women can wear men's jeans if they are over size 32," says Bill Bartlett of E Street Denim in Highland Park, Illinois. "7 For All Mankind's boot cut is a great choice—because of all the stretch in it, it won't make you look like you're wearing men's jeans."

• DON'T CUFF JEANS. Rolled-up cuffs are fattening. Too-long jeans should be shortened at the tailor, no matter what your size.

DRESSING YOUR DERRIERE IN FABRIC
GET THIS RIGHT AND YOU'RE HALFWAY THERE

Fattening Fabrics

THESE UNFORGIVING FABRICS ON YOUR BACKSIDE WILL DO YOU IN.

→ Wide-wale corduroy. Putting a thick fabric like this over an already thick butt is not a good idea.

→ Satin. Shine is not your friend. It reflects off a wide space (your rear).

→ Silk. Not on your behind. It clings to your frame and its thinness will reveal any cottage cheese dimpling. Thicker silks can be flattering, so use discretion.

→ Velour. Especially in a color that pops.

Slimming Fabrics

WEAR THESE, AND YOUR REAR WON'T LOOK AS NOTICEABLE.

→ Cashmere. Light, warm, and terrific layered for coverage.

→ Cotton. Just make sure it's a heavier cotton blend—the key is to stay away from superfine fabrics. Your butt needs structure!

→ Denim. Jeans can do wonders for ample butts; just follow the rules in this chapter!

→ Gabardine. It's tough and tightly woven, so it won't cling to your rump.

→ Lycra® blends. Hold your tush in place and help give it shape.

→ Wool and light wool blends. A great fabric for classic trousers. Buy a pair with a hint of stretch in them for the best fit.

Panty lines on a noticeable butt add insult to injury, so just say no to briefs, bikinis, and girl/boy shorts. If you're not willing to toss out all your panties for shapewear just yet, you might want to keep this challenge on the WIMP (When I'm Mentally Prepared) list. At least toss the ones guaranteed to give you VPL (visible panty line) or more specifically VTL (visible thigh line). While thongs are the best way to get a seamless rear view, they're not the only option. Some other trendy undies to consider are G-strings, tangas, and cheekies.

• G-strings. If you don't mind the feel, these are even skimpier than thongs, so you'll have less chance for VPL.

• Tangas/cheekies/booty shorts. All these terms are all used interchangeably for sexy panties that provide a bit more coverage than thongs. They ride high on the rear and reveal a peek of cheek without the dental-floss aspect of thongs. Better yet when they are seamless. (See Brilliant Buys, page 140.)

BRILLIANT BUYS

BEST JEANS BRANDS

DL1961; Bloomingdale's, bloomingdales.com.

Tory Burch; Nordstrom, toryburch.com.

Adriano Goldschmied (AG); Nordstrom, agjeans.com.

CJ Cookie Johnson; Nordstrom, nordstrom.com.

Citizens of Humanity; Bloomingdale's, bloomingdales.com.

Gap; Gap, gap.com.

J Brand (Bombshell Curvy Fit); Nordstrom, jbrand.com.

Joe's Jeans (Visionaire and Honey); Nordstrom, joesjeans.com.

Habitual; Nordstrom, nordstrom.com.

Levi's; Macy's, jcpenney.com.

Not Your Daughter's Jeans; Bloomingdale's, bloomingdales.com.

Paige Premium Denim (Hollywood Hills); Nordstrom, nordstrom.com.

Rock & Republic; Nordstrom, nordstrom.com.

Seven for All Mankind; Neiman Marcus, neimanmarcus.com.

Victoria's Secret; Victoria's Secret, victoriassecret.com.

JEANS FOR PETITES

DKNY Jeans; Macy's, macys.com.

Banana Republic; Banana Republic, bananarepublic.com.

Jag Jeans; Nordstrom, nordstrom.com.

JEANS FOR SIZE 14 AND UP

Old Navy; Old Navy, oldnavy.com.

Abby Z; abbyz.com.

Eileen Fisher; Eileen Fisher, saks.com.

Paige Jeans; Nordstrom, nordstrom.com.

BUTT-LIFTING SHAPE-WEAR AND TIGHTS

Assets Remarkable Results High-Waist Mid-Thigh Shaper, $34; target.com. Seamless zoned compression and specially-designed rear pockets give the booty an added lift.

Spanx In-Power Line Super Power Panties, style 915, $32; Bloomingdale's, spanx.com. Slims tummy, thighs, rear.

Lipo in a Box Tank Bodysuit, style 46100, $76; lipoinabox.com, qvc.com.

Sculptz Tights, $15; silkies.com. Lifts your rear.

Spanx In-Power Line Super High Footless Shaper, style 912, $28; spanx.com.

CONTROL UNDIES

TC Fine Intimates Edge Microfiber Hipster, style 403, $16; tcfineintimates.com.

NO-VPL UNDIES

MySkins Full-Cut Brief, Girl Short, or Thong, $12; myskins.com. In twenty different skin tones.

Commando Tiny Thong, $22, and Low-Rise Thong, $20; barenecessities.com.

STYLING TRICKS

Instant Button for Jeans, $15; instantbuttonforjeans.com. Just pierce this removable lookalike jeans button through the waistband of your jeans and tighten or loosen the fit up to one-and-a-half inches.

InvisiBelt clear belt in naked, $19.95; invisibelt.com. A thin, flat, lean plastic belt that no one will know you're wearing. No buckle bulge. Also comes in black for black jeans.

Vows *for* Big Booty

- ☐ **I WILL** only wear jeans in dark denim, black, or gray.

- ☐ **I WILL NEVER** wear skirts or dresses cut on the bias.

- ☐ **I WILL NOT** wear pleats of any sort.

- ☐ **I WILL NOT** buy into any of the latest denim trends—clean and simple are best for me.

- ☐ **I WILL** invest in a great-fitting pair of jeans with stretch.

- ☐ **I WILL** donate the tight leather skirts and pants to women with no butts.

- ☐ **I WILL** wear pants in non-clingy fabrics that won't cup my rear end.

- ☐ **I WILL** make sure, when I wear a jacket or sweater long enough to cover my bum, that it's structurally designed to give me an hourglass figure.

DON'T YOU DARE...

Walk around with a uni-butt! Buy shapewear that lifts, separates, and gives you definition back there.

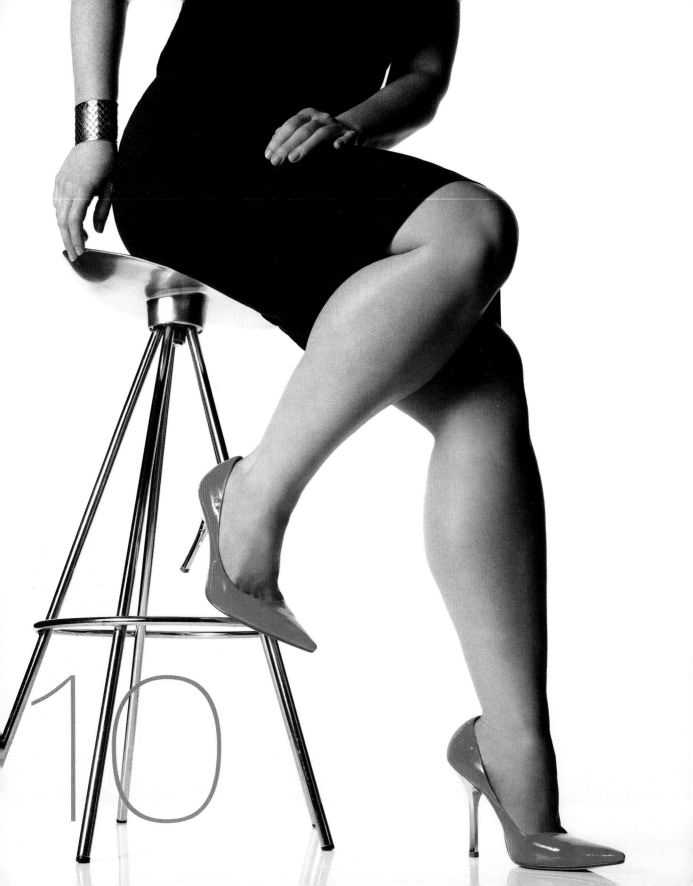

Heavy Calves

YOU KNOW YOU HAVE IT WHEN...

You avoid skirts and dresses . . . You can't zip knee-high boots . . . It's tough getting jeans over your calves . . . Your skirts are all floor length . . . Your calves are as thick as your thighs . . . They measure more than 15 inches around.

→ This chapter is dedicated to all women whose legs have not appeared in public since junior high who, every day, try to hide heavy calves (or varicose veins). Okay, so your legs may never be described as coltish, but is it necessary to condemn yourself to life in pantsuits? Come on. Live a little! Camouflage is a strategy for sure, but it's not the only one. Why not mix it up a bit and also try the strategies of elongation, diversion, and compression? In cold weather, my favorite solution for visually stretching chunky calves is to pair dark opaque tights with slim-fitting dark high-heeled leather or suede boots. Instead of pants, you can wear this boots-tights-combo with a simple sheath and a knee-length coat, or a black dress with a bright-colored structured jacket over it.

This chapter is about exploring your fashion options and breaking out of your particular uniform, whether it's pantsuits, that same tired pair of black pants you always pull out when nothing else works, or even black opaque tights with a slim-fitting black high-heeled boot!

TO WEAR OR NOT TO WEAR LEGGINGS

Fashion purists say that leggings are not for the heavy calved and fat ankled, but if they go all the way down to your ankle—not mid-calf—they beat pasty-white legs popping out from under a skirt or dress. Which brings us to . . .

THE RIGHT TO BARE LEGS

Bare legs can be the sexiest look of all—as long as you're committed to keeping them in top form. If you are going to go au naturel, practice these leg-lifts:

→ SUNLESS TANNING. At this stage, you know how to do this correctly, and when done correctly, self-tanner is a beautiful thing. If you're still gun-shy, start slowly with a build-a-tan formulation.

→ SPRAY-ON STOCKINGS, or bronzing moisturizers, leave an opaque layer of color on the legs, hiding scars and spider veins. The better ones won't transfer onto clothing or come off on your hands. You can't leave home without this, especially on summer nights. Buy it in bulk.

→ GETTING HAIR-FREE. Hairy legs are a turnoff no matter what size your calves are. Remove at your most comfortable price range.

$ The average American woman shaves eleven times per month, according to a study done by Gillette, which is a time commitment, but the cheapest and easiest way to remove leg hair. Second cheapest: waxing at home with a kit.

$$ Get your legs waxed at a salon. Both legs may cost $65 every two months. If you can take the pain, the professional results may be worth it to you.

$$$ If you want to forget about leg hair altogether, laser hair removal in a doctor's office is the answer. You'll need a set of appointments and maybe yearly follow-ups. The average price per one-hour session is $500; for six sessions, $3,000. Hair freedom, for some women: priceless.

BOOT CAMP

Find the Perfect Pair

Stuffing juicy calves into a tall, stiletto boot, desperately trying to close the zipper while the shoe sales associate smiles politely, is almost as mortifying as trying on a swimsuit in a communal dressing room. The horror! Most fashion shoe designers, especially the Europeans, aren't exactly accommodating to the chunky calved. Choosing the wrong boot style can make the difference between Fit Not Fat and Hopelessly Heavy. But sexy, knee-high boots do exist for thick calves, so here's how to find the right pair for your skirts and dresses:

THE RIGHT BOOTS COVER UP THE CALVES and make everything look nice and slim—without cutting off your circulation.

PAY ATTENTION TO COLOR, SIMPLICITY, HEEL, LENGTH, AND FATTENING EXTRAS. Buckles, zippers, bows, grommets, and lace-ups add calories. Think of them as sprinkles, hot fudge, and cherry on the sundae. Do you really need it?

YOU DO NEED A HEEL OF AT LEAST TWO AND A HALF INCHES. Don't fall in love with motorcycle boots or flat boots such as equestrian.

WHERE DOES THE TOP OF THE BOOT HIT? Over-the-knee boots look too lady-of-the-evening. Mid-calf boots and short boots are out of the running, too. Any boot that hits across the widest part of your calf is not the boot for you; it should hit right under the knee.

THE TOP OF THE BOOT SHOULD BE LOOSE ENOUGH TO SLIP A FINGER INTO. Look for boots that can be pulled on in stretchy leather or suede or with elastic panels. As in Stuart Weitzman's 5050 boot, the back is made of elastic and the front is made of soft, buttery leather.

STICK TO DULL, SOFT LEATHERS OR SUEDE; patent is a fattening finish.

YOUR LEGS SHOULD BE THE SAME COLOR AS THE BOOTS. That means, for example, no pale white legs in brown boots. If you have pale white legs, wear brown tights with brown boots. And make sure that they're the same shade—chocolate boots and nutmeg tights can be jarring.

Show your boots some love—they are worth the investment. A shoemaker can make boots look brand new each fall. Get your boots professionally stretched if your legs feel too compressed. You can have a special elastic panel added to a pair of boots that no longer zip. "So many people just throw eight-hundred-dollar boots into the closet," says New York podiatrist Suzanne Levine, DPM. "They spend so much money on boots, yet they're cheap when it comes to using boot trees to retain the shape."

A CALF-FRIENDLY GUIDE TO
SKIRTS / DRESSES / PANTS / STOCKINGS / SHOES

SKIRTS AND DRESSES

Yes, you can wear skirts and dresses. You don't have to hide your legs under ankle-length skirts just because of your calves. Knee-length A-line skirts and dresses may give you the best look, particularly if you're petite. Hemlines that hit mid-calf or right above the calf need to be shortened. Skirts that taper in at the calves, need to be shortened or to go away. Also, get rid of skirts with slits down the back, a veritable peep show for the back of your calves!

PANTS

Flared black pants are your most flattering cut and color. Buy two pair so they can be in heavy rotation. Wide-leg pants elongate the leg. I know it's hard to wrap your head around, but wide-leg pants won't make you look wide. Just as skinny pants won't make you look skinny if you aren't. Skinny pants = fat. Wide pants = thinner. Skinny jeans or tapered pants will cling to thick calves, making them all the more obvious. Exhume from your closet any and all jeans and pants that taper in below the knees.

STOCKINGS

It's more youthful to go without pantyhose in the workplace. That said, for a column I wrote for *More* magazine on the subject, I interviewed women in corporate America who deemed nude pantyhose an absolute essential from nine to five. Not because of a mandatory dress code, but because it makes them feel more professional, more in control. If you feel more confident wearing pantyhose, stick with the nude hose, but know that you have options. Black opaque tights are the most universally flattering hose on everyone. But whatever dark color you wear, make it similar in tone to the dress or skirt you're wearing.

Don't choose hose too thick. Check the dernier on the package (the number that measures sheerness). The smaller the dernier number, the finer the material is. Ultra-sheer hose, usually dernier 15 or below, is best for evening wear. Dernier 15–30 work for work, 30–40 are semi-opaque, and 40 and higher are full-on opaque. The higher the dernier number, the thicker the hose will be, so don't go above a dernier 40, as it will bulk you up.

When it comes to added extras, such as diamante detail, stay far away from them, as well as any stockings with seams down the back. Larger-net fishnets can cut into your fleshy calf, making the fat poke out (not an attractive look!). Fishnets are nonfattening when the netting is very small. You can't buy a better pair of fishnets than those by Spanx—small nets, yes! And a control top that gives a nice, sexy bottom and alleviates grid butt, yeah! To look Fit Not Fat, stick to black, navy, or dark brown nets. Did you know that professional dancers wear a pair of sheer, thin hose underneath the nets? It makes the skin underneath look perfect while also preventing your toes from poking through. Just in case you were thinking of competing in *Dancing with the Stars!*

SHOES

The right shoes are all about creating a perfect balance. Dainty shoes when paired with heavier calves can look disproportionate—like you're trying to stuff yourself into something made for a doll. Same goes for ultra-skinny stilettos. A heel of an inch or higher will visually lengthen your legs, but be careful the heel isn't too pencil-like—the contrast of a thin heel only accentuates thickness in the calves. Color counts, too. For summer, when you go barelegged, the must-have is shoes the same color as your leg: nude for pale legs, tan for darker legs. Some Fit Not Fat shoe guidelines:

Clunky shoes make calves and ankles look clunky. So beware of the wedge heel.

Round and square-toed styles are fattening—they shorten your foot.

Booties so popular these last few seasons, even with skirts, take inches off legs.

A slim pump with a pointed toe is the nonfat shoe of choice. But petites look dwarfed in too pointy a toe.

Double ankle straps are double fattening—one ankle strap is fattening enough.

10 THINGS THAT MAKE YOU LOOK FAT WHEN YOU HAVE
Chunky Calves

1. **A neon-colored stocking** with a shoe bootie—the fashion equivalent of mac and cheese

2. **Pasty legs in a chunky platform sandal**

3. **Calf overhang on a mid-calf boot**

4. **Dark hairy legs**

5. **Super-skinny 7-inch stilettos**

6. **Leggings in any color other than black**

7. **Standing with your legs kissing**, instead of one leg slightly in front of the other, with the front toe pointed at a 45-degree angle

8. **Clam digger pants with ballet slippers**

9. **Skirts or pants with crazy patterns or in garish colors.** Small floral prints, big floral prints, and busy Lilly Pulitzer and Pucci prints can be fattening.

10. **An asymmetrical dress with flip-flops**

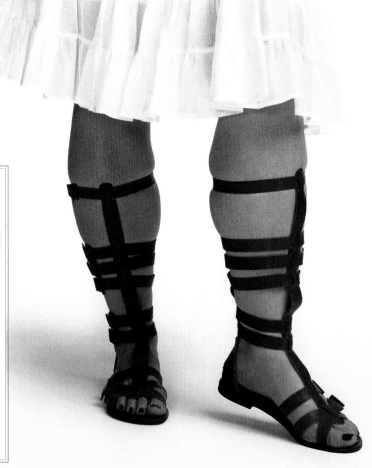

....

HIGH FAT:
Gladiator sandals are
a recipe for disaster . . .
horizontal straps across
the widest part and heels
as flat as pancakes. Make
this trend ancient history.

HOW FAST CAN YOU
GIVE THESE AWAY?

HIGH FAT

× Calf-length boots; furry après-
ski boots

× Capris or harem pants

× Bright or light-colored tights

× High gladiator sandals

× Large windowpane fishnets

× Roll-up cuffs on jeans

HIGH FAT *vs.* NO FAT

→ Alright, we stacked the deck a bit, but can anyone look at this and say that shoes and stockings
don't really matter?!

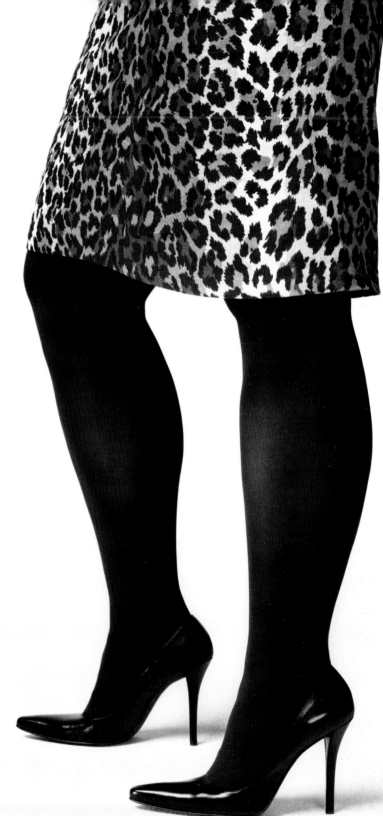

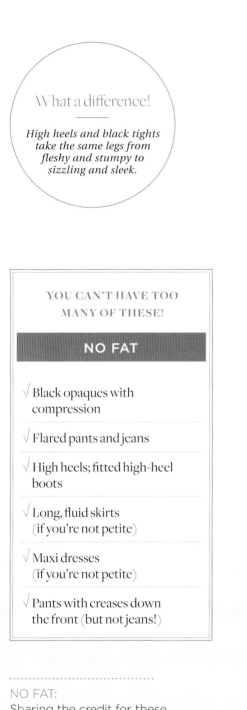

What a difference!

High heels and black tights take the same legs from fleshy and stumpy to sizzling and sleek.

YOU CAN'T HAVE TOO MANY OF THESE!

NO FAT

√ Black opaques with compression

√ Flared pants and jeans

√ High heels; fitted high-heel boots

√ Long, fluid skirts (if you're not petite)

√ Maxi dresses (if you're not petite)

√ Pants with creases down the front (but not jeans!)

NO FAT:
Sharing the credit for these shapely gams: A pointy toe and a 3-inch-plus stiletto. A round or square toe is just not as leg lengthening.

Thinner by Tonight!

INSTANT GRATIFICATION

Shave your legs.

Shorten your mid-calf skirt to the knee.

Compress the calves with black control tights.

Kiss the Crocs good-bye.

Step into black opaques and knee-high black suede boots.

Self-tan your legs or spray on "stockings."

Throw on a pair of fabulously sexy pumps or high-heel sandals— they'll draw eyes to your feet and away from your calves.

Going to Extremes: *Cosmetic Leg Procedures*

Cosmetic leg procedures could easily be mistaken for torture techniques. Calf-reduction and leg-lengthening surgeries, mostly performed in Asia, are risky and painful and fall under the category of "No way in hell!" The scary news is that calf-obsessed women are getting Botox injections in their calf muscles. (Is there nothing that Botox isn't used for?) The Botox atrophies the calf muscle, which, in turn, slims it out. The downside: You may experience temporary paralysis in the calf. They better come up with something else, because this just isn't worth the risk.

VEINS
Obvious veins are no fun, and paired with fat calves, they pack a double whammy. But both spider and varicose veins are common complaints. "By age fifty-five, 50 percent of women will be affected by varicose or spider veins," says New York dermatologist Deborah S. Sarnoff. Spider veins are the tiny magenta bursts of broken blood vessels, while varicose veins are those bulging, ropy looking things you can feel with your fingers. Genetics are by far the biggest factor on deciding if you'll be one of the unlucky 50 percent, but lifestyle plays a part, too. "Pregnancy, bumping your legs a lot, standing for long periods, and habitually crossing your legs all stack the deck against you," says Dr. Sarnoff. Wearing compression stockings, such as those by Jobst (compressionstore.com), will improve your circulation and may prevent additional veins from forming, but what can you do at the doctor's office to remove the obvious veins you already have?

OPTIONS FOR SPIDER VEINS
1. Sclerotherapy. A tiny needle is used to inject the vein with a chemical agent. The vein collapses, and over a period of weeks, the body absorbs the now nonfunctioning vessel and clotted blood, and then they simply disappear. The typical treatment will have several tiny injections that last about 15 minutes. After the injection, the area is compressed with either support hose or pressured dressing. There's little downtime. Rare occurrences are temporary hyperpigmentation and cramping.

2. Laser therapy is used if the vessels are too tiny to get the needle into. The same lasers are used that treat broken blood vessels on the face. The overlying skin is protected, while the vessels are zapped through the skin. When the beam of light is delivered, it's attracted to the hemoglobin, which is in the blood. The light is converted into heat and seals the vessels and collapses the blood vessel wall and eventually the body absorbs it again.

OPTIONS FOR LARGER VEINS AND VARICOSE VEINS

1. Ultrasound-guided foam sclerotherapy (UGFS). A liquid sclerosing agent is mixed with air in the syringe to make it foamy. The advantage to having it bubbly is that it enhances the duration of contact with the venous wall and is more likely to stay in the area it's injected. As with all of these treatments, compression stockings are worn one to six weeks afterward. The likelihood of serious side effects depends on the amount of foam injected. You don't want to exceed more than 10 cc's per session. Downside: possible hyperpigmentation.

2. Endovenous laser therapy (EVLT). The area is blown up with anesthesia and then a laser system is passed through a hollow needle into the vein. Once it's in the vein, the needle is removed, like starting an IV. Energy is delivered to the vein in the form of light. After activation the laser is

SWAP-OUTS:
WAYS TO HIDE THE HEFT

Instead of	→	Go for
Asymmetrical dress		An A-line dress
Clunky platform wedges		Pointy-toe mules
Cropped pants		Wide-legged pants
Lacy patterned tights		Solid black opaque tights
Leggings as pants		Pants as pants
Leggings that hit mid-calf		Leggings that hit at the ankle
Miniskirts		Maxi skirts
Neon tights		Black, navy, brown, or gray tights
Patent leather boots		Soft leather boots
Rolled-up jeans		Boot-cut jeans
Shoe booties		Knee-high heel boots
Skinny jeans		Trouser-cut jeans
Slouchy suede boots		Slim-fitting, knee-high heeled boots

pulled back continuously. Downside: There's a possibility of burning the outer layer of skin and a less than 1 percent risk of deep vein thrombosis (blood clot).

3. Radio frequency ablation (RFA) Radiofrequency waves heat up the inside of the vein and collapse it. Local anesthesia is used, and the doctor feeds a probe inside the vein. Little twitches of pain in the area of treatment may last for several weeks. There's also a possibility of skin burns and inflammation. ●

BRILLIANT BUYS

LEG BRONZER

Sally Hansen Airbrush Legs (in 5 shades), $9.95; mass retailers, drugstore.com.

Laura Mercier Body Bronzing Makeup, $38; Bloomingdale's, Sephora, lauramercier.com.

DuWop Revolotion SPF 15 Bronzing Body Moisturizer, $28; Sephora, sephora.com.

EXFOLIATORS

Yes to Carrots C the Body Carrot Rich Moisturizing Body Scrub, $9.99; mass retailers, target.com.

Neutrogena Energizing Sugar Body Scrub, $9.99; mass retailers, drugstore.com.

MOISTURIZERS

Yes to Carrots C Through the Dry Spell Deliciously Rich Body Butter, $12.99; mass retailers, target.com.

Clinique Deep Comfort Body Butter, $24.50; Bloomingdale's, clinique.com.

Neutrogena Deep Moisture Butter Body Cream, $8.10; drugstore.com, mass retailers.

RAZORS

Gillette Venus Embrace 5-Blade Disposable Razor for Women, $12.99; mass retailers.

Gillette Venus Bikini Kit (Venus Embrace razor, Venus Bikini trimmer, Olay Bikini lotion), $10.79; mass retailers.

SHAPERS

Lipo in a Box High-Waist Capri, style 46852, $49; lipoinabox.com. Leg shaper with open gusset for bathroom ease.

TC Fine Intimates Even More Pantliner, style 4317, $56; for stores, see cupidintimates.com. Smoothes from waist to butt to calf with the Wonderful Edge hem so it won't ride up under tight pants.

LEGWEAR

L'eggs Profiles Benefits, waist smoother toner sheer energizing hosiery, style 93763, $8.99; Wal-Mart, cvs.com. Sheer hose on high-waist shapewear.

L'eggs Profiles Opaque Tights, energizing leg, $8.99; Wal-Mart, cvs.com.

Sculptz Shapewear Sheers, $12.50; silkies.com.

Spanx High-Waisted Tight-End Tights, style 167, $28; spanx.com.

Spanx High-Waisted Tight-End Tights—Control-Top Fishnets, $28; spanx.com.

Spanx Tight-End Tights—Convertible Leggings, style 039B, $32; spanx.com.

Spanx High-Waisted Tight-End Tights, $38; spanx.com.

SHOES

Fit Flop Walkstar III, $58; fitflop.com. They claim to help strengthen and tone calves. Whether they do or not, they are easier to walk in than your ordinary unsupportive flip-flop!

Stuart Weitzman 50/50 boots, $595; stuartweitzman.com. These slightly over the knee boots with a one-inch heel have an elastic panel to ensure a great fit.

Vows *for* Leggings

- [ ] **I WILL** only choose a pair that ends at the thinnest part of my ankles.

- [ ] **I WILL NOT** wear leggings in place of pants, with a big top or sweater, even if the said big top or sweater covers my butt.

- [ ] **I WILL** only wear leggings in no-fat colors such as black and brown and navy and gray, not red, orange, yellow, green or blue.

- [ ] **I WILL NEVER** wear leggings in white, cream, or ivory.

- [ ] **I WILL NEVER** wear Crocs, clogs, or sneakers (yes, even Keds) with leggings.

- [ ] **I WILL NEVER** wear ribbed or lace-edged leggings—too fattening—even if they're Wolford.

DON'T YOU DARE...

Wear shoe booties or short boots with skirts or dresses, even if you're wearing black opaques. It's like chopping yourself off at the knee.

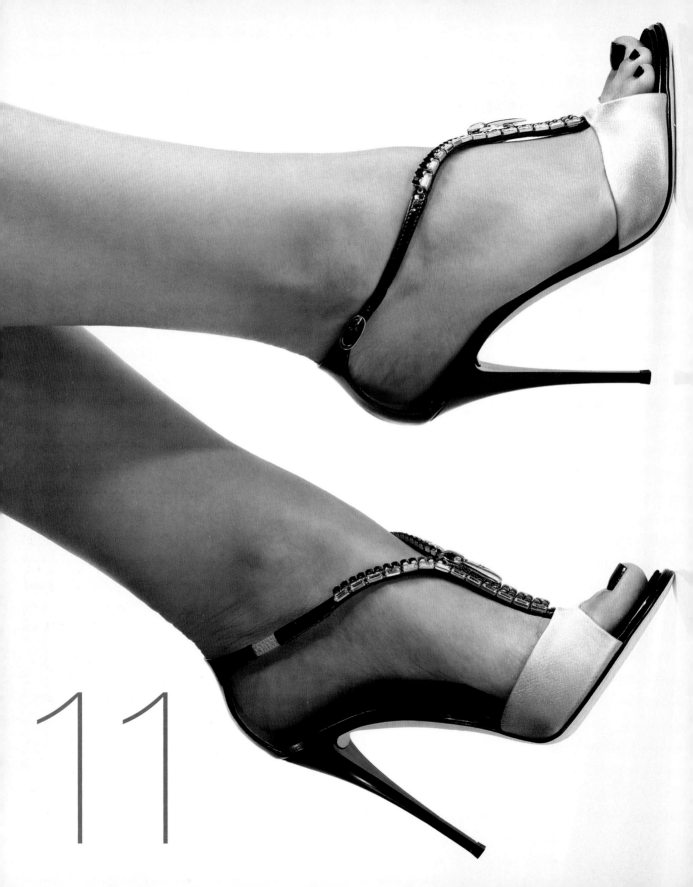

11

Wide Feet + Ankles

AKA
duck feet, claw foot, club foot, hobbit feet, fat ankles, chubby lower legs, cankles

YOU KNOW YOU HAVE IT WHEN...
Ankle bracelets don't fit, ever ... Your calves are the same width at your knees and at your feet ... You have bunions, corns, or hammertoes, and maybe all three ... Your mother's legacy is wide feet, and yours are starting to look like hers ... You wish there was such a thing as beach boots.

→ Remember when we were kids, and we would get our feet measured every time we went shoe shopping? Do you remember putting your foot into that metal sliding device? When was the last time you had your foot measured? Do they even have a foot-measuring device in your favorite shoe department? They don't at Barneys New York, where I have bought many a shoe too small for me. But I can't blame Barneys for the fact that I still assume that I'm the same shoe size that I was thirty years ago. The truth is, our feet flatten (widen) and lengthen with age. If you were a size 6 at twenty, then you should be in a size 7 at fifty, says Dr. Suzanne Levine, the New York podiatrist who has made it easier for many famous feet to strut the red carpet. Our feet spread as a result of normal aging, according to Dr. Levine, but did you know that weight gain can account for a larger shoe size? I always thought that the reason for our shoe obsession was because no matter how much weight we gained, we would always,

always fit into our shoes! Well, not true! So how can we get our feet to look thinner and smaller?

"You can lose weight in your feet if you lose overall body weight," says Dr. Levine. "Perfect example is during pregnancy the feet get wider. After pregnancy, the swelling goes down." Which is why, after having a baby, you should get your feet measured again, as you may have gone down a shoe size. "Obese people have heavy feet," says Dr. Levine. "A lot of it is just fluid retention. Once you lose weight, you're not retaining as much fluid in the feet."

So, if you have wide feet, you can either lose weight or wear shoes that downplay your feet and make them less of an issue. And, if you have cankles, which are heavy-looking ankles, you can minimize their impact on your overall look by camouflaging them in boots or pants and diverting all eyes to your more fabulous features—eyes, shoulders, neck, cleavage, waist, rear, wherever. ●

for Wide Feet+Ankles

Clothes are so voluminous that the Fashion Gods are giving us chunky shoes to balance them out. Caged heels, shoe booties, ankle-strap platform wedges, sculptured heels, seven-inch heels... topped with metal, charms, gems, and buckles... If you haven't bought these shoes yet, don't.

→THE STRATEGY IS ALL ABOUT selecting shoe styles that flatter your foot. A slim, pointy shoe with a spindly heel will draw attention to a wide foot—and the contrast between the shoe and the foot will make the foot look fatter. But a wide foot in a thick, clunky platform wedge will make your foot look chunky. The solution? A moderate shoe, such as a graceful, feminine peep-toe pump, with a thick but curved heel, would balance out a wide foot and heavy ankle.

At this moment in fashion, because the clothes are so voluminous, the Fashion Gods are giving us chunky shoes to balance out the big top, the A-line dress, and the sculptured jacket. The edgiest shoes are the ones that will make chunky feet look their chunkiest. Fashion magazines are filled with knee-high gladiator sandals, caged heels in neon-bright patents, Oxford-tied shoe booties, ankle-strap platform wedges, sculptured color-blocked heels, and stacked seven-inch heels. As if these fetish styles weren't fattening enough, designers have topped them off with embellishments, such as thick metal edging, gold logo charms, hardware and grommets, candy-colored jewels, high-shine buckles, ladylike bows, glitter, tassels, and fringe!

"Simple styles are going to be more elegant and flattering," says Nancy Boas. "The shoe should have the elements of bareness, but it should be covered enough to mask some of the imperfections."

If you haven't bought any of these shoes yet, don't. There is no point in buying into a trend that doesn't pay off for you. If you have, well, no one wants to throw out shoes that she just bought. Next season, you'll edit these styles out of your life, but until then, put them into your get rid of WIMP file.

From now on, only buy comfortable shoes that will make your feet look thinner and smaller. My friend Nancy Boas, the accessories (shoe) editor at *Glamour* when I was beauty director, went on to design shoes for Nine West and is now vice president of design for women's shoes at Ralph Lauren Collection. She knows firsthand what styles look best on real (not model) women. "Fashion and flattering don't always go hand in hand," she admits. "At the end of the day, you want your legs to look sexy and shapely." According to Nancy, "Most difficult to wear are sandals with multiple, wraparound straps, such as gladiator sandals— they're for women with skinny legs. If you don't have perfect legs, you need to take into consideration how many straps you have around your ankles. Straps around the ankles cut off the leg, they make the leg look shorter, and they make your ankles look heavier." The strategy is to find shoes that keep the ankle unencumbered as much as possible.

"Simple styles are going to be more elegant and flattering," says Nancy Boas. "The shoe should have elements of bareness but covered enough to mask imperfections." Worth trying: the peep toe, which is more covered than a sandal, but shows a little toe cleavage, always sexy.

If it's a bunion that's making your feet look wide, you need to buy shoes that subtly camouflage it. Find a shoe as bare and as clean as possible but that covers all the right places. "It needs to have enough straps that go straight across the bunion. On some strappy sandals with tiny feminine straps, the bunion will push through. Just make sure that your toes don't pop out the sides."

What else works? Actually, there are lots of ways to make your tootsies feel better. On the next page is the list to take with you next time you're shoe shopping. ●

NOTE: *Don't go shoe shopping in the morning.*
I have a friend who loves to be the first in the mall on Saturday. At ten o'clock she practically opens the place, because she doesn't like fighting the crowds later in the day. It took her years to catch on to the fact that when she did buy shoes, it was early in the morning. When she put on the same shoes in the evening, her feet were swollen, and the new shoes were tight and painful. Learn from her experience! Buy shoes later in the day when your feet are their biggest.

SHOES THAT MAKE YOU LOOK FAT WITH
WIDE FEET + ANKLES

Let's think twice before we take these home again.

• GLADIATOR SANDALS, ESPADRILLES, MARY JANES, AND ANY OTHER SHOE WITH ANKLE STRAPS. "Straps around ankles cut off the leg, they make the leg look shorter, and they make your ankles look heavier," says Boas.

• PENNY LOAFERS, OXFORDS, DRIVING SHOES. Any shoe that looks like it belongs in a man's closet should not be in yours, as it won't do your foot any favors. Clunky, masculine shoes need to be in a soft leather and in a delicate shade, like camel. Otherwise, they look too masculine.

• CLOGS. Crocs, which technically are a clog, have replaced Uggs as the new ugly "it" shoe. Don't go there. Any kind of clog-like shoe is going to make you look fat and sloppy. You might as well wear a sign reading, "I've given up!" And no, it doesn't matter how many charms you stick in the holes to jazz them up.

• FLATS. Save them for times you need to be super-comfy (e.g., running errands, walking around town). Also, don't think you're doing your feet any favors by wearing flats; they offer no support to the heel and arch and can lead to painful plantar fasciitis, says Dr. Levine.

• BIRKENSTOCKS. No matter how many times these come back in style, take a pass. Doubly nerdy when worn with socks—ew.

• FLIP-FLOP SANDALS with a wide piece of horizontal fabric over the toes will make your feet look wider.

• SHOES EMBELLISHED WITH BOWS, BUCKLES, BUTTONS, OR SEQUINS. Why add bells and whistles onto a foot that doesn't need any?

• SQUARE OR ROUND TOES. Both extremes shorten and broaden your feet. Moderately round is better than moderately squared.

• FIVE-INCH (OR MORE) SPIKY HEELS. On a petite, they look like you're on stilts. On a larger woman, they look out of proportion; a stacked high heel works better.

• SHOES IN HIGH CONTRAST COLORS AGAINST THE LEG. Black shoes on pale legs look fat! Brights are more fattening than neutrals.

• WHITE SHOES. Unless you're a nurse, and even then, see if you can get around this. Neutrals are so much chicer.

• KITTEN HEELS. These petite, low heels are not ideal for those with heavy ankles or calves. The proportions may look off as the scale of the kitten heel is tiny.

• SNEAKERS! Traditional clodhopper white lace-up sneakers worn outside of the gym are super-fattening. Do you have to wear sneakers on the street? If so, choose a pair that are sleek and cool, more about style than athletic performance.

WHY SO MANY REALLY CUTE SHOES
DON'T FIT A WIDE FOOT
And What to Do About It

An informal poll of friends revealed that we are only wearing 10 to 20 percent of the shoes we own. (Want to see how universal this is? Ask a few of your friends what percentage of their shoes they are actually wearing. See if you get the same results.) Why aren't we wearing the other 80 percent? Some shoes are kept for decoration purposes only, slightly out of style but they add pizzazz to the shoe collection. Okay, but the rest? They kill us, every time we put them on, in one place or another.

Why do so many really cute shoes hurt? Do this bit of homework, and you'll see for yourself. Measure the widest part across your entire foot (it may be from bunion to bunion). Then, round up all the shoes you aren't wearing. Measure the toe box across the width of the shoe, the section that contains the widest part of your foot. Most high-fashion shoes have a three-inch toe box. My foot measures three and a half inches across. And I wonder why these shoes K-I-L-L. Many women have feet that measure four inches across, an entire inch bigger than most fashion shoes!

Two truths that keep wider feet from enjoying the cutest shoes: 1) A fit-model for shoes has perfect feet. If her feet got wider due to pregnancy, age, or weight gain, she would be out of a job! Bunions, hammertoes, corns, and calluses are her occupational hazards. So if the shoe fits her perfectly, what is the likelihood that it will fit you? 2) High-fashion shoe designers (such as Manolo Blahnik) tend to keep their widths very narrow because that's the aesthetic of the brand—thin and elegant like the women who wear them.

Now that we know what the problems are, let's work around them. For starters, you might be more comfortable in shoes that use a European fit—it's slightly wider. "Certain companies subscribe to an American fit, and others go with a European fit. And there's no real way of knowing who uses what, so you have to try everything on," says Nancy. "The standard fit measurement is 6B for American sizes, and European standard is 37B-C, which generally blends the width between a B and a C." There are brands right now that are on the forefront of melding comfort and style. The Italian brand Geox, for example, does shoes with a 3¾-inch toe box.

Also, don't be embarrassed to get measured or to bring your own measuring tape with you. "Shoes are like bras: They're so technical and they really have to fit," says Nancy. "The absolute worst thing you can do is buy shoes that don't fit—even if you love them." Even if they're on sale. We've all been to shoe sales when the prospect of scoring a pair of Chanels, Choos, Blahniks, or Louboutins for one-third or more off is just way too tempting to pass up, so we try to cram our feet into bright, shiny shoes that simply do not fit. If the shoe doesn't fit in the store, it doesn't fit. If you remember nothing else from this chapter, remember that. Why do we believe that once we get them home, something magical will happen in our shoe closet to make them stretch? Sales associates who think nothing of egging you on by uttering the lie, "They'll stretch out," should be called on the shoe carpet. What they're really saying is that your bones and soft tissue, over time, will rub against the leather until it gives. Ouch! That's how we get unsightly bunions, corns, blisters, and hammertoes. Thanks a lot.

A FOOT-FRIENDLY GUIDE TO SHOES

―――――

These styles will keep you standing tall.

d'Orsay heels

The number one most flattering shoe for women with cankles. This style is open on the sides and can have either open or closed toes; slingbacks or closed backs. "They don't break the line of the leg," says Nancy. "So the legs look really long."

Ankle boots

Not to be confused with shoe booties, low-cut ankle boots under jeans and pants, will be more comfortable than higher ankle boots or knee-high boots. They look very fashion forward worn with dark opaque tights under skirts and dresses if you have slim calves.

Knee-length boots

Wear under skirts or dresses. The tucking-jeans-into-the-boot trick only looks good on Hannah Montana and friends. Just make sure your boots have a heel if you want a no-fat look.

Flesh-toned or nude pumps

You can't have enough flesh-toned shoes in warm weather. Buy these in leather, patent, or snakeskin. A simple pump with a sexy, elegant line that matches your skin tone is a great way to elongate your leg.

Peep-toe pumps

A pedicured toe is an easy way to show a little sexiness and draw attention to the toe, away from the ankle.

Mules

Terrific for summer and year-round in warmer climates if the vamp is low and doesn't cut across the ankle to make you look fat. A two- to three-inch heel is universally flattering.

Stacked or chunky heels

Good, chunky, curved heels will make your ankles look thin in comparison, but not overwhelm the foot. Just make sure they're not on big, fat platforms, which will make you look fat.

Slingbacks

Sexy! They keep the ankle clean, which equals skinny. Many women (including me) love the slingback look but complain about slippage. If this is your problem, too, check out the adhesive strip from Foot Petals. It's the answer for this common problem.

Wedges

An easier way to get taller than wearing heels. If you've sworn off skinny heels, do give a moderate wedge a chance.

PRETTY FEET DON'T LOOK FAT

If you have short, wide feet, an easy way to deflect unwanted gazes is to keep them neatly pedicured with a light or sheer polish without a lot of fuss (no crazy colors, no nail art). To save money, learn to do your own pretty pedicure at home. Dr. Levine does, to ensure her own medical standards of cleanliness—then she goes to the salon for polish. If you do go to the nail salon, it's smart to bring your own nail files, cuticle clippers, orange stick, brushes, or even your own pedicure kit to prevent fungus and whatever else could be growing there!

Now, About Your Toenails...

→ The length and shape of your toenails will make a difference, says Essie Weingarten, founder and president of the beloved nail polish line Essie Cosmetics, who recommends that toenails hit the end of the skin. "If you have a heavier leg, keep toenails more square than rounded and a little bit on the longer side."

→ Choose a chic, sophisticated neutral toenail color, such as sheer pink or beige.

→ Dry, cracked heels make a fat foot look worse. In the shower, pick up a pumice stone to exfoliate the dry skin on your heels.

→ When you come out of the shower, slather on thick moisturizer and slip on cotton socks. Letting the cream settle in for at least an hour will help smooth and soften dry, cracked heels.

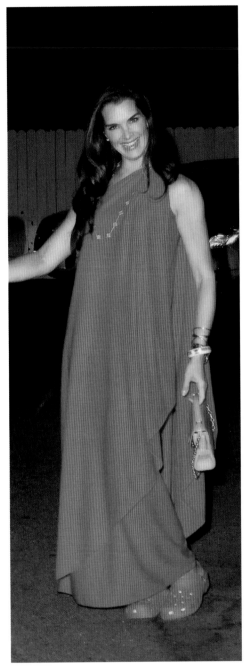

Crocs for evening? Er, no. Even if you look like BROOKE SHIELDS, even if you may be recovering from foot surgery, footwear doesn't get any more fattening than a pair of pink crocs.

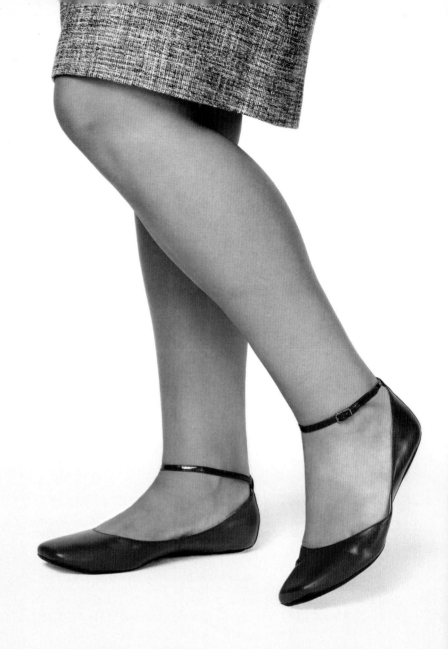

HIGH FAT:
The flatness of this shoe doesn't help, but wearing an ankle strap is like drawing a circle around the problem—here, in bright red.

HOW FAST CAN YOU GIVE THESE AWAY?

HIGH FAT

× Ankle straps

× Clogs, Crocs

× Flats of any kind

× Round and square-toe pumps

× Sneakers

HIGH FAT *vs.* NO FAT

→ When dressing a cankle, the next best thing to boots is a naked ankle in a classic high heel. Yes, flats are more comfy, but try to slip on a heel at least when going out, so you won't look dumpy and frumpy.

NO FAT:
Keep the ankle bare in a high heel in the same shade as your leg; by elongating the leg, you'll look taller, thinner, better.

YOU CAN'T HAVE TOO MANY OF THESE!

NO FAT

√ d' Orsay pumps

√ Flesh-toned heels

√ Mules

√ Peep-toe pumps

√ Slingbacks

Thinner by Tonight!

INSTANT GRATIFICATION

Match your shoes to your leg color; not to your skirt or dress. A monotone color all the way down will lengthen the leg. In winter, wear a black opaque stocking and black pump; in summer, skin-toned slingback with bare legs.

Compress cankles with longer-length footless shapewear such as Spanx's Under the Heel Tight-End Tights, a support hose for women with bloated ankles. The top part extends beyond the ankle to the top of the foot; the bottom slips under your heel. You don't want to wear anything that cuts across your ankle at its widest part.

Slip on a pair of d'Orsay heels (see page 162). Add cushiony support from a gel pad to make them comfy.

Wear a boot-cut jean or wide-leg trouser rather than a harem pant or cropped pant that ends before the ankle. Pair the slightly flared pant with a stacked heel or wedge instead of ballet flats. The idea is to keep your cankle under cover.

Give away your foot jewelry; ankle bracelets and toe rings are attention-getters, so who needs them?

When it comes to shoes, why do we believe that once we get them home from the store, something magical will happen in our closet to make them stretch?

REASONS TO TREAT YOUR FEET
LIKE PRECIOUS JEWELS

Wearing uncomfortable shoes that don't fit you well is a vicious cycle you don't want to get into. The more times you wear shoes that don't fit you properly, the more damage you'll end up doing to your feet. Foot surgery is a big deal and should be avoided at all costs. Want to prevent your feet from getting fat—and ugly—going forward? Treat them like precious jewels, today.

BUNIONS. Beware of a very pointed toe. Pointy-toe shoes make the foot look longer, thinner, sexier . . . but too pointy can bring on bunions. Yes, bunions are hereditary, but wearing shoes that are too tight around the toes can provoke them, according to Dr. Levine, who says, "I never met a bunion that didn't have a pointy shoe in its history." If your mother has bunions, do yourself a favor and start looking for more moderate pointy-toes from now on. Even if your mother doesn't have bunions, if you can't resist a pointy-toe, try one size up to give yourself more wiggle room.

THE PUMP BUMP. If you trot around town in shoes that don't fit, you up your chances of developing other funky foot deformities that will make your feet look bigger, longer, or wider, such as "pump bump" (aka Haglund's deformity), hammertoe, corns, calluses, and blisters. Pump bump is a painful, swollen heel bump from pump-style shoes rubbing against the heel. If you have this, see a podiatrist. And look for backless shoes such as mules.

HAMMERTOE is a smaller toe that bends down abnormally and may occur when a too-long toe is continually forced into a cramped toe box. Corns or callouses, which are also brought on by shoes that are too tight and narrow, can form over the hammertoe joint.

MORTON'S NEUROMA, an enlarged nerve that usually occurs between the third and fourth toes, is an excruciatingly painful cramp that "freezes" your feet or toes into an uncomfortable position. It often occurs when you're lying down, after a day of walking around in a too-tapered toe box or extreme high heels. It's your body reminding you that you need a wider toe box and to limit the amount of time in high heels. In other words, don't commute to work in them; wear more comfortable shoes for transportation.

Why Cankles Aren't Funny

Everyone's laughing about cankles. There's even a jokey Web site, saynotocankles .com. The word *cankle* comes from calf + ankle and describes an ankle that has no definition, one that's almost as wide as the calf. This chapter is about how to disguise fat ankles, but if your ankles are abnormally swollen, and you are not pregnant, you really need to see your doctor. Ankle edema could be the result of weight gain, it could also be too much sodium or signal more serious medical issues. Better to get checked out.

Going to Extremes: *At the Podiatrist*

Your podiatrist can custom-make you a pair of orthotics so you can wear heels more comfortably. These aren't inexpensive (prices start at $250). There's a slim chance your health insurance may cover them. A plaster cast is made of your foot to get the size and the arch just right, then it's sent out to be made into a rubber sole that you can slip into your boots, closed shoes, or peep-toes. You can't wear them in open-toe sandals because they'll show. And some shoes might be too small to accommodate them. But when they work, they're great.

As we age, the fat padding that cushions our soles begins to diminish, making the wearing of stilettos even more painful than before. If money is not an issue, you may want to consider getting a syringe of Juvederm or Sculptra injected into the bottom of the feet to restore volume. This is high maintenance, for sure, but women who stand on their feet all day, such as flight attendants, are doing it.

BRILLIANT BUYS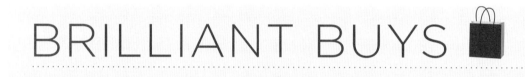

SHOES

TKees (T-keys) Flip-Flops to match your skin tone, $44; Bloomingdale's, tkees.com. If you have to wear flats, these—in leather or suede—will at least make your legs appear longer.

SHOE PAD BRANDS

Kushyfoot.com

AirPlus for Her; target.com.

Dr. Rosenberg's Instant Arches; instantarches.com.

Dr. Scholl's for Her; mass retailers or beauty.com.

Foot Petals; footpetals.com.

MOISTURIZERS

Udderly Smooth Foot Cream with Shea Butter, $6.49; mass retailers, drugstore.com.

Heel Magic, $12.95; hsn.com.

Burt's Bees Coconut Foot Crème, $9; mass retailers, drugstore.com.

Aquaphor Healing Ointment, $5.99; mass retailers, drugstore.com.

PEDICURES

Essie in Petal Pink, Pop Art Pink, Knockout Pout, Playa del Platinum, Jazz, $8 each; Ulta, drugstore.com.

OPI Nail Lacquers in I Pink I Love You, I'll Take the Cake, Passion, Makes Men Blush, At First Sight, Rosy Future, Rumple's Wiggin', $8.50 each; Ulta.

Miss Oops Pedicure in a Bottle, $18; missoops.com.

PedEgg, $10; pedegg.com.

Tweezerman Pedicure Solutions 7-piece pedicure tool kit, $50; tweezerman.com.

Tweezerman Pedicure Ceramic File-Ice, $20; tweezerman.com.

Vows *for* Wide feet

☐ **I WILL NOT** wear shoes with ankle straps.

☐ **I WILL** carry a pair of comfier (yet still chic) shoes with me when wearing stilettos.

☐ **I WILL NOT** get a French pedicure or sport any sort of toenail art.

☐ **I WILL NEVER** wear open-toe shoes without a pedicure.

☐ **I WILL NOT** show toe cleavage that looks like the flesh is spilling over the shoe.

☐ **I WILL NOT** wear sandals with straps that pinch and strangle my toes.

☐ **I WILL NOT** let peds show.

☐ **I WILL NEVER** wear sneakers with a skirt.

DON'T YOU DARE...

Settle for ugly comfort shoes when you can find stylish ones that feel just as good.

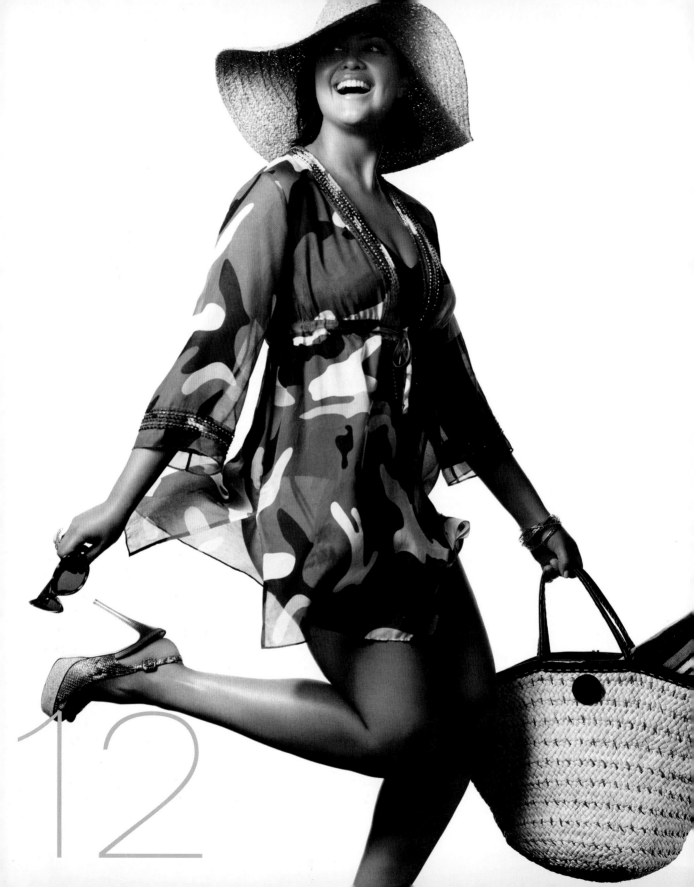

Summer

YOU THINK YOU LOOK FAT IF...

You don't own a swimsuit . . . You do own a swimsuit but can't remember the last time you wore it . . . Sundresses and shorts scare you as much as the words "bring a swimsuit" . . . You decline invites to beach and pool parties that sound like fun . . . Nothing would make you set foot in the swim department of any store . . . Regardless of the heat, you always wear a jacket and pants for maximum coverage . . . You can't wait till Labor Day when summer is pretty much over.

→ If there's one season that strikes fear into grown women, it's summer. Because if you're not happy with your body, you're not happy from Memorial Day to Labor Day. Of course, if you live in the Sun Belt, you experience the hell of summer all year long. When the temperature soars, you want to strip down to nothing, but you can't. You can't let everyone see you half naked. Well, it's not that you can't—you won't. Because it's too humiliating. You would rather suffer in hot cover-ups than reveal your body in public. I hear you. I have been there. It may make you feel a teensy bit better to know that almost everyone reading this has been there! Why do

you think that January is the biggest month for diet and exercise? Because we're all trying to look better by the deadline—Memorial Day, the unofficial start of Show Your Body Season. For those of us who live in colder parts, where it's sometimes still chilly at the end of May, we have a little cushion of time, say, until July 4th, when everyone begins to notice that we are not baring our arms and legs like everybody else.

Even though summer is, without question, the most challenging time of the year to hide fat, it's not impossible. You'll be so much happier about the season once you learn a few tricks. All you need are some smart strategies for covering up that won't look as conspicuous as a pair of black capris and a long, black button-down shirt on the beach when everyone else is in swimwear.

So let's collectively take a deep breath. We're going to do this . . . we're going to look as Fit Not Fat as we possibly can. Don't you dare miss out on all the fun because you don't want to be seen in a swimsuit. If you let that happen, the weight terrorists win! Here's to your thinnest summer ever. ●

YOUR DRESS-THINNER STRATEGY
for Summer

THREE NEW SUMMER UNIFORMS

1) Instead of wearing the same dark pants and jackets that you wore day in, day out the rest of year, let's lighten up for the season in style. If you love pants and your butt is not your problem, choose white or khaki and pair them with a crisp tunic. Add the highest sandal that you can walk in, plus a hoop earring and a stack of bangles and you're good to go. Tory Burch is the designer responsible for bringing back this sixties-style tunic. There's a new one from her each season in different prints and embroidered trims, and it often becomes the best seller in every collection. Why do women love the tunic? "It's an incredibly flattering silhouette," says Tory. "Over a skinny pair of jeans, it looks elegant, and it's so forgiving. For someone who isn't in the best shape she's ever been in, the tunic makes her look elegant and smooth." You can find tunics now everywhere and at every price point. Even at Chico's!

2) When you're not wearing a tunic, and you need a layer of warmth in overly air-conditioned offices, movie theaters, or airplanes, invest in summer-weight cashmere V-necks or long cardigans in yummy colors. Layer over body-shaper camisoles, bare tops, or dresses.

3) A third easy summer option is a fresh dress in a pretty pattern. One zip, and you're done. You don't have to worry about tops and bottoms. Add the same accessories—high strappy sandal, a hoop earring, a stack of bangles—and you're about to embark on a no-fat summer.

When you're not wearing a tunic, and you need a layer of warmth in overly air-conditioned offices, movie theaters, or airplanes, invest in summer-weight cashmere V-necks or long cardigans in yummy colors. Layer over body-shaper camisoles, bare tops, or dresses.

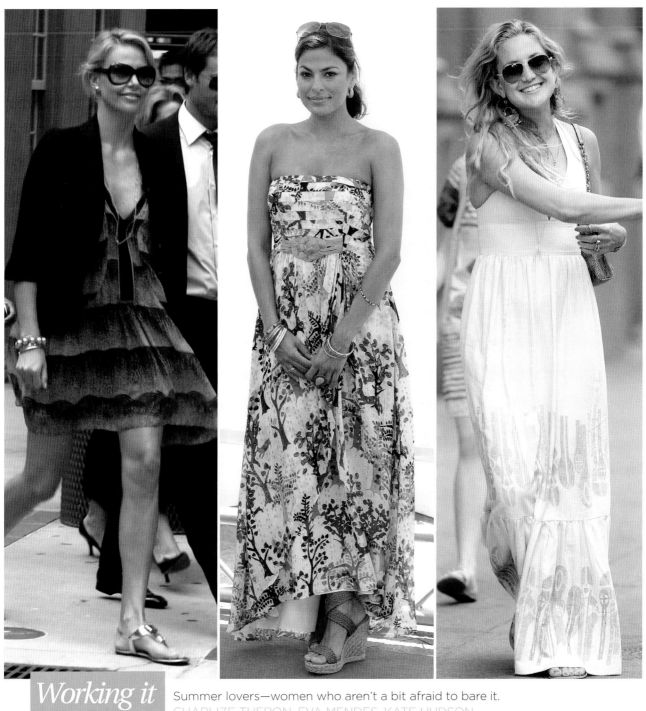

Working it

Summer lovers—women who aren't a bit afraid to bare it.
CHARLIZE THERON, EVA MENDES, KATE HUDSON

SHOPPING FOR A SWIMSUIT

This is by far the most humiliating part of summer. I remember when I was more overweight than I am now, trying on swimsuits in a department store dressing room and being so depressed staring at my out-of-shape, pale, flabby body. I'm sure you can relate to the experience of standing there almost naked in the dressing room. Once you peel the too-tight suit off, you don't want to get dressed again to search the racks for a larger size. You have to beg a sales associate to come to your rescue. And you just wait there until she turns up with the size. There's a comedy sketch in this all-too-common female experience, but really, what a waste of time. And what is the deal with the dingy lighting? And do they search for brutal mirrors? If you really wanted to test drive the suit, you'd have to parade around in front of total strangers. Even though my weight issues today are different than they were before, the ick factor of that experience still lingers. I no longer try on swimsuits at stores. I just can't do that to myself.

So how does one buy a swimsuit today with dignity intact? Online. I know that you are probably thinking that there is no way you would do that, but let me explain. Go to a few sites that have fabulous swimsuits—even your favorite retailer online. Order three of every suit you want: your size, then one size up and down. Throw a try-on party for yourself one night or on a Sunday afternoon. Be sure to de-fuzz your legs, get a bikini wax, and do a self-tan and a pedicure before you attempt this, because you want to look your best in the three-way mirror (or two mirrors that allow you a good back end view). Try on your swim accessories, too. You can use a clothing rack, if you happen to have one, and if not, use your bed to lay out all your possible cover-ups, such as tunics, blouses, sundresses, sarongs plus sandals, sunglasses, and a big floppy hat, so you can evaluate your complete look.

You might want a glass of wine to get you in the mood or put on some of your favorite music and relax. Before removing the tags, road test the suit at home, doing all the things you could never do in that cell of a dressing room. Sit, lie down, bend over, try on different shoes, lift your arms to be sure you won't fall out, pretend swim, do a cartwheel, jog around the bedroom. Make sure you're in love with the suit. Once you decide upon the keepers, ship the rejects back with UPS, FedEx, or the post office, and you're done! You might want create a new ritual for yourself—a launch party—to get yourself physically and emotionally ready each summer before you go public.

SECRETS FROM THE SWIMSUIT DRAWER

I live in swimsuits on weekends during the summer. I put on a swimsuit and cover-up and wear it around the house all day, thinking there might be a moment when I actually go out and read in a lounge chair. Of course

---

Pull together a total look for swim.
Looking polished from your sun hat to your sandals boosts your confidence when you need all the confidence you can muster. Don't just settle for any old baseball cap, flip-flops, beach bag, and ratty old towel or sheet. Take the time to coordinate all your accessories, and you'll look and feel better. Not just better, hot, in the best sense of the word.

A BODY-FRIENDLY GUIDE TO THE
10 BEST BLACK SWIMSUITS

Little black dress, little black swimsuit. Black is the most slimming color, so why not give yourself the best shot at looking your slimmest? Women are so convinced that covering up is the ultimate solution they sometimes look for the biggest piece of black fabric they can find. They overdress the body with a huge swimsuit, covering up more than they actually need to. But the truth is that not everyone needs to wear a one-piece. There are plenty of hard-bodied women in their forties and fifties who may want to mix and match two pieces, as very few women are the same size top and bottom. If you have the bod, it's better to wear a two-piece than a tankini, which has a way of rolling up and showing more than you intended to. The ultimate black swimsuit should be as much of an essential as your everyday T-shirt bra.

Classic wide V-neck tank
The number one universal flatterer—wide V balances hips, thighs, and derriere; elongates and balances body

Shirred or draped suit
Fabric is softly gathered to flatter and hide muffin top and belly

Power suit
Body-shaper control compresses to shave pounds

Empire or raised-waist suit
Shifts emphasis from tummy and thighs to the chest

Crossover tank
Carves a waist and hides jiggly midriff

Printed suit
Allover florals, animal prints, swirls, or artsy patterns can strategically blur bulges—or not

Strapless
Highlights toned shoulders and arms and balances a broad tush, hips, and thighs; get the newest with molded bra

One shoulder
Sexy coverage and elongates the torso so your breasts don't sit on your waist

High-waist bikini
Controls bareness, hides tummy

Halter
Adjustable neck lifts and shapes large breasts

that moment rarely comes, but still, I have a lot of very comfortable suits and some look better than others.

You cannot buy a suit without trying it on. Over the years, I've bought suits at Super Saturday—a madhouse designer yard sale in the Hamptons to benefit the Ovarian Cancer Research Fund. There are no dressing rooms there in the middle of the horse farm, so unless you want to strip down to your undies in front of the world, forget about trying anything on. If you have less than a model body, taking a chance on a suit without trying it on is a big mistake. A zebra-striped suit that has horizontal stripes across the tummy—what was I thinking? A gold metallic one-strap with no shelf bra? How old did I think I was—twelve?

Why not buy a shapewear swimsuit? The new kid on this block is Spanx. If you want to look slimmer at the beach or pool without sacrificing an ounce of chic, these suits are for you. They compress just like their beloved shapewear but look cool, and are on trend and in fashion colors. Miraclesuit Swimwear started this trend and claims to take an inch off your waist. Its suits

WHERE TO SWIMSUIT SHOP ONLINE

Victoriassecret.com, Newport-news.com, Landsend.com, and LLbean.com allow you to mix, match, and build your own swimsuit. For women who wear two-piece suits and require different size tops and bottoms, these sites give you the freedom to customize size, style, and color. You can take a size 14 bottom and a size 10 top, or you might want to choose a darker bottom and lighter top to draw the eye upward instead of down. LLbean.com has a "Live Help" link.

Nordstrom.com has a fantastic chart of the latest suit trends.

Everythingbutwater.com offers a Fit and Style Guide plus the chance to make an appointment to meet with a swimsuit fitter at one of its retail stores. For women with fit issues, navigating the waters of swimsuit shopping online can be treacherous, so your life raft might be a specialty store, such as Everything but Water, with a sales staff trained to fit swimsuits, and nothing but swimsuits, all year long.

> If you have less than a model body, taking a chance on a suit without trying it on is a big mistake.

really do measure up. I actually took a tape measure to my waistline before and after. Another brand is Magicsuit, from victoriassecret.com, in some styles to size 16DD.

WHY YOU NEED A HOT COVER-UP

It's smart to put as much effort into your cover-up as you do your suit—maybe even more. Because if it's a little chilly outside or you've decided not to take the plunge, you may never take the cover-up off! Some people don't see your suit, just your cover-up. That's why you may want to consider buying a new cover-up every year, even if you don't buy a new suit.

10 THINGS THAT MAKE YOU LOOK FAT IN *Summer*

1. Wearing all black.
If it's not depressing you, it's depressing everyone around you. Mix it up a bit with white or a pastel. Don't make your inability to go with the light spirit of summer so obvious.

2. A daily uniform that hides your body.
Shapeless black knit pieces abound, and so do deadly pull-on pieces with elastic waistbands and S-M-L sizing. Mix relaxed and fitted pieces; show some skin and body definition with V-necks, a skinny belt at the waist, and elbow-length sleeves.

3. Getting so summerized that you forget to dress strategically.
Wear all the Lily Pulitzer pinks, greens, corals, and florals you want, just keep necklines, proportions, and color breaks in mind. This is not the time to plunge into boob-baring halters, ankle-wrap platform wedges, and tissue-thin tees that show back fat!

4. Wearing a tankini and thinking no one knows that you're trying to hide a tummy.
Either wear a two-piece and show your middle or get a shapewear suit with a tummy-control panel. Tankinis don't work because they have a tendency to ride up—and expose you.

5. Letting your boobs hang out in a tank top, tee, or swimsuit without a built-in bra.
Just because you're spending a casual weekend lounging around the beach or doing errands is no reason to go unsupported.

6. Squished bosoms and too much cleavage.
Stopping short of the nipples is a big no. Slip dresses and itty-bitty sundress tops or triangle bikinis are ridiculous after a certain age, even if you're in St. Tropez. What if you run into someone you know? Better to go for a wide V neckline or a one-shoulder look. Sexy, not slutty.

7. Spillage at the top or sides of a swimsuit or tank.
You don't want to look like you gained a few pounds after you bought it. Swimsuit brands such as Sunset Separates, La Blanca, Anne Cole, and Tommy Bahama are great for bigger boobs, and some offer bra sizing for full coverage.

8. Metallic swimsuits or shiny satin skirts just invite trouble.
Shine accentuates every bulge and squiggle, no matter how great it looks in glossy fashion magazines. A gorgeous gold satin pencil skirt or a silver swimsuit will catch the light in all the wrong places. Stay matte or textured when it comes to fabrics, or just add your shine in accessories—like a few bangles or metallic sandals and tote.

9. Swimsuit leg openings that are too low, too tight, or too binding.
Low-cut legs on a suit looks matronly no matter how sexy the neckline. Look for laser-cut suits with no bindings, modified higher leg lines that won't dig into the fleshy part of your hip. Start an inch below the hipbone as the highest point of the leg opening—it works for most women.

10. Shorts and boy short swimsuits.
I know they are enjoying a surge, but honestly, short shorts are only for teens, and boy shorts suit women with boyish, narrow figures. They cut right across your leg at the widest part in a straight horizontal. Not what we need.

HIGH FAT *Vs.* NO FAT

→ The same rules apply to swimwear. Horizontal stripes make you look fat, especially when there's not enough of them to go around. And, accessories are essential to create a bold fashion statement. PS: Don't forget the sunless tanner—it will make you look like you've dropped a size!

HIGH FAT:
Itsy bitsy teeny weeny pink and white striped bikini lets it all hang out, exposing too much boob and muffin top.

HOW FAST CAN YOU GIVE THESE AWAY?

HIGH FAT

× Baggy grandma-skirt suits

× Bikinis

× Cutout swimsuits

× Extreme-plunge necklines (to the waist)

× Metallic swimsuits

× A neck-to-toe caftan

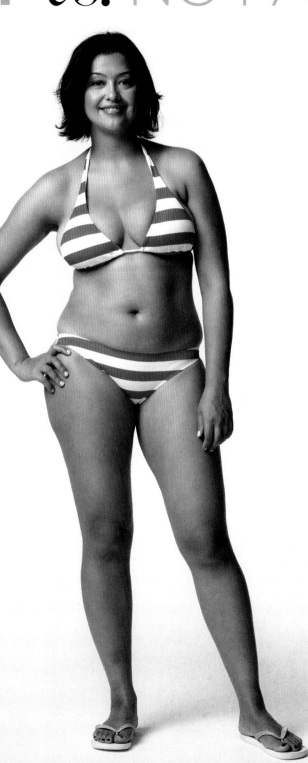

YOU CAN'T HAVE TOO MANY OF THESE!

NO FAT

√ Dark, oversized sunglasses

√ Halter-style necklines

√ Hoop earrings

√ Ruched suits

√ Shapewear suits

√ Strapless suits

NO FAT:
Yes, it really is a miracle suit! A dark V-neck ruched one-piece subtracts inches and adds confidence. You want a suit that controls like shapewear.

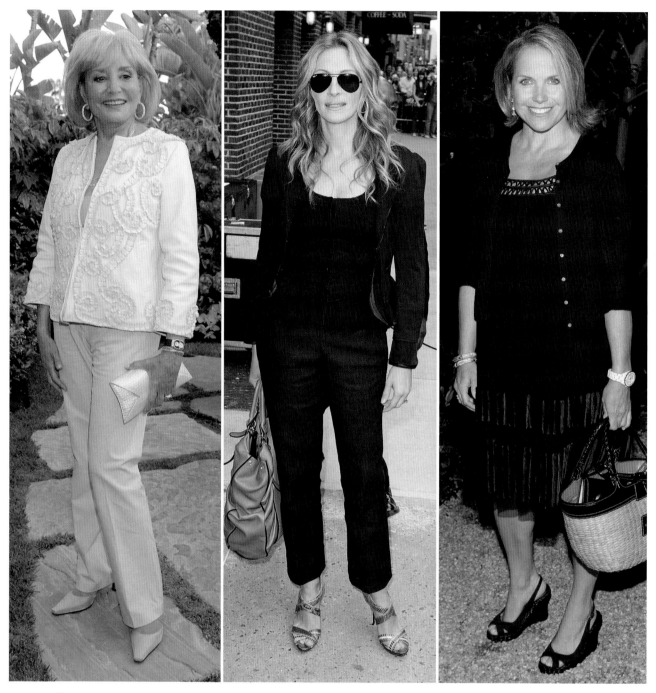

Effortless summer chic is an outfit that looks professional and polished without resorting to a matchy-matchy business suit. Look Fit Not Fat in summer: wear separates in a unifying monotone color, show some skin at the neck, and keep yourself long and lean in a shoe with height.
BARBARA WALTERS, JULIA ROBERTS, KATIE COURIC

HOW TO NEVER LOOK FAT IN A COVER-UP

An oversized T-shirt doesn't fool anyone. It's easy, but it's also high fat and prevents you from looking Fit Not Fat at the beach or poolside.

A lightweight sundress over your suit can give you coverage and look chic. I bought an Indian-print spaghetti-strapped empire-waist one at Topshop, but you can also find them on the racks at Forever 21, H&M, Zara, Target, JCPenney, or any major department store.

A sarong will work if you tie it without adding bulk at your hips, which is tricky (see Tying a No-Fat Sarong, right). The secret is to buy one in a soft, matte, very lightweight printed fabric—the lighter and more handkerchief-like the better— because it's easier to tie and won't add an extra inch of fabric around the lower body where we need it least. The print makes it opaque and hides cellulite. Next time you're vacationing on a tropical isle, start collecting sarongs. I love the ones from the store Calypso, and they last for years! ●

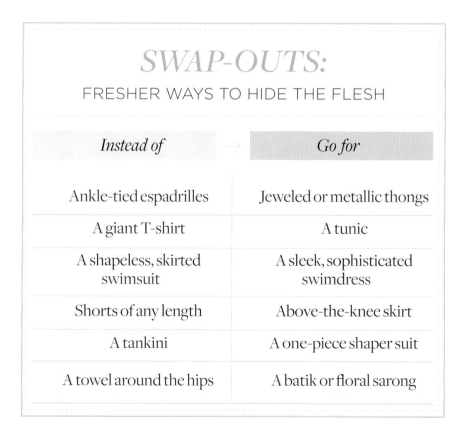

SWAP-OUTS:
FRESHER WAYS TO HIDE THE FLESH

Instead of →	*Go for*
Ankle-tied espadrilles	Jeweled or metallic thongs
A giant T-shirt	A tunic
A shapeless, skirted swimsuit	A sleek, sophisticated swimdress
Shorts of any length	Above-the-knee skirt
A tankini	A one-piece shaper suit
A towel around the hips	A batik or floral sarong

TYING A NO-FAT SARONG

Unwrap the sarong so that it is a full rectangle—not folded.

Place the middle of the sarong at your behind (as if you were wrapping yourself up in a waist-high towel).

Grab the top two points of the rectangle, then move your hands in along the top edge of the fabric toward you, about halfway between the end point and your body.

Bunch the fabric up on either side of you, so you have what looks like two fingers of fabric.

Double-knot both those fingers together, close to the body just below your waist.

Take the dangling top end of one side and tuck it under the top of the fabric, across your belly and into the waistband under the knot.

Let the other end fall free in graceful folds. This will look so much less fattening than the heavy swaddling that most women do.

Thinner by Morning!

Self-tan.

If you have a light skin tone, getting a spray tan at a salon or doing your own smearing the night before can hide all those things that shouldn't see the light of day—like veins, cellulite, stretch marks, and brown spots. If you're darker skinned, you're ahead of the game.

Get a swimsuit with built-in body-shaper compression.

They can whittle your entire body down a size and provide lift at the bosom and rear so you look like you spent the year spinning and doing Pilates. And if you slip your body-shaper suit under a tunic or sundress, you'll look slimmer in that, too!

Make V's not boxes at your neckline and thigh.

V-neck halters in tops, sundresses, and swimsuits are guaranteed transformers that elongate the body. Straight low boy-leg suits and minis that cut your upper leg at the widest point form a boxy shape that makes your rear and thighs appear huge.

Create a diversion.

A print with a lot of movement can blur body flaws, and so can shirring or draping. Swimsuits are 90 percent illusion, 10 percent coverage, so take advantage of these strategically placed details. The same applies to beach cover-ups, tops, and dresses.

Start at the neckline—to balance proportions.

A halter or wide V in a swimsuit, dress, or top creates a power neckline that flatters a big bosom, draws the eye away from your tummy, and balances hips and thighs. A strapless swimsuit or empire cocktail dress with a molded bra can do the same.

Watch your back.

A very low scoop back can make a big booty seem less so.

Be cheeky.

Let a little cheek show in your swimsuit. Full complete butt coverage is matronly! It can also make your behind look bigger than it is. Modified coverage—not dental floss—is the idea.

Buy as close to your dress or pants size as possible when it comes to swimsuits.

Going up a size or two to fit into a suit makes your bust and rear droop—you won't be getting the support you need.

SUMMER SOLUTIONS

IF YOU'RE PETITE…

• STICK TO ONE-PIECE SUITS AND SUNDRESSES WITH ONE STANDOUT DETAIL—maybe a bow at the neckline of a strapless suit or a ruffle down the front of a suit. But not bows, ruffles, shirring, and print all in the same piece.

• KEEP SWIMSUIT NECKLINES AS LOW AS POSSIBLE, leg lines as high as possible to stretch the body. The more chest and upper thigh you show, the better.

• WEAR HIGH SHOES like wedges or platforms or mules—not flat flip-flops—to keep the look lean and leggy.

• TUNICS WILL WORK AS KNEE-LENGTH SUNDRESSES. Look for dense opaque colors even in lightweight cottons and jerseys.

• DO YOURSELF A FAVOR AND CHECK OUT SWIMSUITS DESIGNED FOR PETITES, IN STORE AND ONLINE. Landsend .com, for instance, offers their slimming SwimShape suits in petite sizes.

IF YOU'RE SIZE 14 & UP…

• LEARN TO LOVE TUNICS. Paired with white pants, you have your summer uniform. Long pants look better than capris.

• CHOOSE THE WIDEST V-NECKLINE in swimsuits, tops, and sundresses to give your upper body a powerful inverted-triangle shape.

• LOOK FOR LONG CAFTANS AND STRAPLESS ANKLE-LENGTH EMPIRE SUNDRESSES for tasteful poolside cover rather than shorter styles. This only works if you're tall and can pull it off.

• TRY WRAP OR SURPLICE WAIST SUITS, SUNDRESSES, AND TOPS that create or emphasize a waist for definition.

• LOOK FOR AN ALLOVER RUCHED SUIT WITH FIRM CONTROL SHAPING in a sexy style that will contour your curves, not hide them.

• SEE THE SHOPPING RESOURCES IN SKINNY CLICKS (pages 239 and 242), as an increasing number of up-scale retailers are now catering to larger women for swimwear and everything else. (It's about time!)

BRILLIANT BUYS

SWIMWEAR BRANDS

Norma Kamali (normakamali collection.com) Ruching and flattering '50s style.

Shape fx (barenecessities.com) Shapewear-focused swimwear for all target spots.

Carmen Marc Valvo (bloomingdales.com, victoriassecret.com) Silky fabrics and goddess draping.

Gottex (saksfifthavenue.com, bloomingdales.com) Best selection of wide deep V-neck suits in prints.

J. Crew (jcrew.com) A rainbow of colors and high-quality fabrics.

Lands' End (landsend.com) Contemporary full-coverage suits.

La Blanca by Rod Beattie (bloomingdales.com) One-shoulder suits that sizzle.

LL Bean (llbean.com) Great basic tanks and suits with UPF (Ultraviolet Protection Factor of 50+) sun protection in suits.

Magicsuit by Miraclesuit (nordstrom.com) Super control brand up to 16 DD.

Michael by Michael Kors (Bloomingdale's, macys.com) Rich-looking suits with luxe details like hardware, bows.

Miraclesuit (Bloomingdale's, barenecessities.com). Sucks up fat and holds it in till you take it off.

Shoshanna (nordstrom.com) Flirtatious suits with cup sizes up to DDD.

Spanx Swimsuits (Bloomingdale's, spanx.com) The biggest splash in the swimwear department in years. There are sexy one-piece deep-V halters that are anything but matronly, trendy bandeau and one-shoulder suits with ruffles, even flirty swim dresses. No fussy patterns, just slimming solids in colors that are sublime: lavender, teal, black, and red. Suits range from $150 to $200, and sizes 4 (in some styles) to 18 (in some styles).

SUNSCREENS

La Roche-Posay Anthelios 45 Ultra Light Sunscreen Fluid with Cell-Ox Shield, SPF 45, $27.90; laroche-posay.us.

Neutrogena Sunblock Lotion Sensitive Skin SPF 60, $10.99; mass retailers, drugstore.com.

Neutrogena Ultra SheerBody Mist Sunblock SPF 70, $9.99; mass retailers, drugstore.com.

Clinique Sun SPF 50 Face Cream, $17.50; Bloomingdale's, clinique.com.

Shiseido Sun Protection Liquid Foundation SPF 42, $34; Bloomingdale's, bloomingdales.com.

SELF TANNERS

Xen-Tan Transform Luxe Premium Sunless Tan, $30; Nordstrom, nordstrom.com.

Jergens Natural Glow Firming Daily Moisturizer and Revitalizing Daily Moisturizer, $8.99 each; mass retailers or drugstore.com.

Tan Towel Half Body Classic 15-pack; $19.95, hsn.com.

Clinique Self Sun Body Tinted Lotion, $20; Bloomingdale's, clinique.com.

Vows *for* Summer

- ☐ **I WILL** buy at least one lightweight tunic.

- ☐ **I WILL** give up my illusions of string bikinis and get a sexy one-piece.

- ☐ **I WILL** stop talking about my weight and select shaper suits and shirring.

- ☐ **I WILL** make sure that I have a great cover-up for every suit.

- ☐ **I WILL** take advantage of lightweight summer sweaters.

- ☐ **I WILL** have at least one killer black suit I can rely on.

- ☐ **I WILL** cut out the size tag and not freak out anymore.

- ☐ **I WILL** give up my belly ring.

- ☐ **I WILL** accessorize swimsuits as I do all my clothes—with stylish shoes, jewelry, sunglasses, and a hat.

DON'T YOU DARE...

Go topless. Your breasts need support. Plus, do you really want to risk getting basal cell carcinoma on one part of your body that hasn't been exposed to a lifetime of sun?

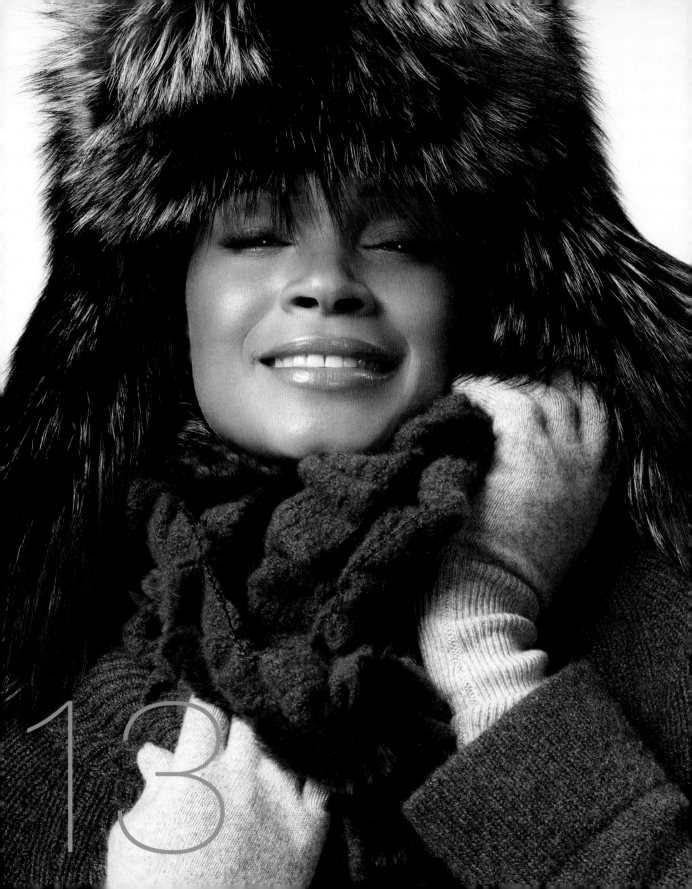

Winter

YOU THINK YOU LOOK FAT IF . . .

You can't get your seat belt across in the car . . . You appear ready for hibernation . . . Your boobs and butt make hills and humps under your coat . . . You cannot wear a hobo or shoulder bag with your coat on . . . You look forward to winter as a haven for hiding from the world.

→ For the last six months, all the women in my neighborhood look like they belong to the same tribe, snapped into longish black hooded puffer coats that have all the shape of a sleeping bag. The belted versions with vertical quilting aren't quite as fattening as those with horizontally stitched packets of down padding, but all puffers more or less bulk you up like the Incredible Hulk. If you're reading this book, you shouldn't have a knee-length puffer in your closet. Don't let a coat do you in. There's no time like the present, so go ahead, put this book down, and bag that coat up for your city coat drive! (Find one near you on onewarmcoat.org.) Now congratulate yourself for losing twenty pounds so fast!

I grew up in Chicago, where I've never been colder, so trust me when I tell you that in the right coat, it is possible look slim and sleek in freezing temps without getting frostbite. If you haven't bought a new coat in two to three years, it's time to go coat shopping. In the coat section of your favorite department store, you will find a dizzying selection in vibrant colors, quirky patterns, belted, pelted, with three-quarter sleeves, lush cuffs, bold shoulders, nipped-in waists, and long, lean silhouettes designed to give a better body. In the old days, the conventional wisdom was that your coat should last forever, so your wool classic in black, navy, or beige was simply replaced when it got shabby. Now you're witnessing the result of a

If your coat is the only thing people see you in for seven months of the year, it will inform that first impression. Why be forgettable in a boring basic when you can wow everyone in a memorable coat loaded with personality? Bring on the color, the shine, the pattern, the drama! This is one bleak season where we definitely need some extra fashion fun!

seismic shift in designers' attitudes toward the coat, putting the fun back into functional and creating fashion statements that make us never want to say "coat check."

Having just one coat these days is as sad as having just one bra! Michelle Smith, designer of one of my favorite brands, Milly, made the flashy coat with metallic threads that brought me many compliments last season. She once told me, "Multiple coats are essential for the grown-up wardrobe." She suggests at least four, depending upon your lifestyle needs—a tailored black coat with luxurious detailing for work, a solid-color to wear with jeans, a glamorous cocktail coat, and a faux or real chubby (stole) for dressy evening. It makes sense to have a few of varying lengths. Just FYI: There was once a rule that said skirts should not stick out from a coat. Forget that. You'll look hipper if your skirt is either a little longer or quite a bit longer than the coat.

(I hope that made your day!) Slipping on one of these new coats, as I once said in my "Fashion Grown-Ups" column in *More* magazine, is the most fun you can have with your clothes on!

The coat as fashion item is welcome news for women in colder climes in need of a psychological lift to survive the season. We snow bunnies live in our coats from October to April (that's about 210 days; more than half the year). At the movies, in restaurants, at concerts, and in the mall, some of us never remove our coats! If your coat is the only thing people see you in for seven months of the year, it will inform that first impression. Why be forgettable in a boring basic when you can wow everyone in a memorable coat loaded with personality? Bring on the color, the shine, the pattern, the drama! This is one bleak season where we definitely need some extra fashion fun!

If I haven't convinced you to buy a

new coat yet, consider the economy. Spending your fashion dollars on a special coat is a wise buy because it dresses up whatever basics you already own. A fashion coat doesn't just make your outfit; it is your outfit . . . That's why it really doesn't matter what you've got on underneath, because who sees it? So if you want to buy just one thing this fall, get yourself a coat that makes you look Fit Not Fat. ●

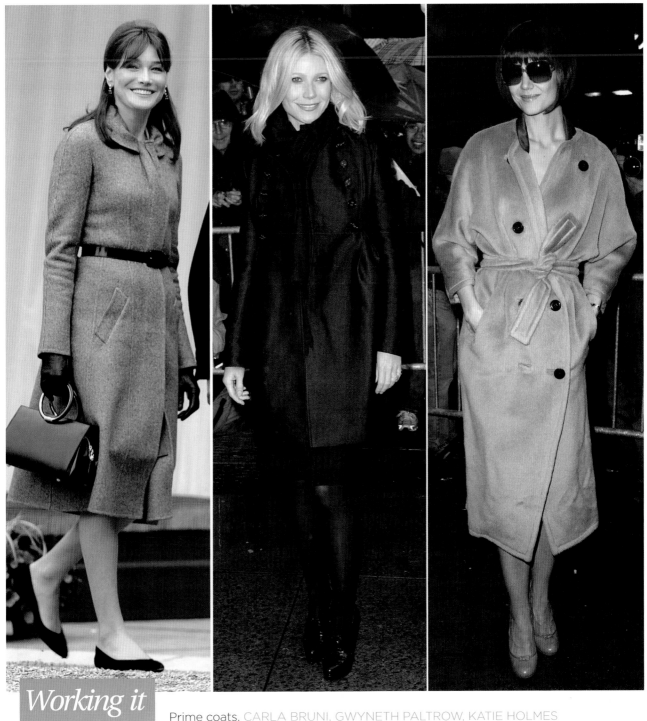

Working it

Prime coats. CARLA BRUNI, GWYNETH PALTROW, KATIE HOLMES

YOUR DRESS-THINNER STRATEGY
for Winter

→ IF YOU DON'T ANALYZE the fat content of your winter coat and accessories, bundling yourself up can add serious bulk to your frame. Start with the lightest coat you can get away with, because you want to layer. But it's not about just piling on more layers like you're making lasagne. Winter calls for strategic swaddling.

What works and what doesn't in a winter look? One that doesn't is a perpetual favorite of fashion magazines: Julie Christie's overly romanticized *Dr. Zhivago* look. You may recall the image of her wading through snowdrifts in a ground-sweeping military-inspired coat trimmed in fur, all along the hem? Don't try this at home unless you're six feet tall and don't have to drive a car or hail a cab. Puddle-sweeping coats make most women look like grubby extras from a period movie. Maxi winter coats shorten you and make you look dumpy, not to mention how filthy they get crossing city streets.

This winter, the coat of the season is the casual belted bathrobe. If you're at all heavy, it's going to be hard to keep that belt tied, and a big knot atop the menopot? Right under the bust? This style coat slices the short-waisted into two distinct upper and lower body chunks. So instead, let's embrace the coats that will make us look Fit Not Fat.

BE PICKY WHEN SHOPPING FOR A COAT

The fabric, shape, cut, shoulders, length, scale, proportion, color, trim, accessories . . . every detail of the coat matters. So let's make sure all these details are working for you and not against you.

BE PICKY ABOUT LENGTH

Most women look best in a knee-length coat—no longer. Ankle-length maxi coats reappear as a trend every so often and look dramatic on six-foot-tall models on a runway. If you're five-foot-four or under and you wear a maxi coat or even an ankle-length coat, you will lose out on the chance to show your legs. Showing leg elongates you . . . it's a major body booster. Remember that shorter knee-length coats worn over skirts with boots will have you looking longer and slimmer than mid-calf coats worn over pants, always.

BE PICKY ABOUT SHAPE, STRUCTURE, AND FIT

A boxy, shapeless coat makes you look bigger than you really are. A structured coat with oversized shoulder pads will make you look like you've dug up your Pat Benatar look from the '80s; and if you're short and top-heavy, you'll look like you're going to fall over. Choose a coat style that fits your widest area and your smallest, too. Women with big boobs who are smaller in the shoulders don't need extra shoulder width. Women with a big booty need the ease of a back vent or a coat that has enough volume on bottom, but they may not need that volume on top.

BE PICKY ABOUT FABRIC

The wider the garment, the more fluid the fabric should be—coats with full bell-shaped skirts, bathrobe styles, drop-waist pleats, and blousons, should all drape gracefully. Cashmere, silk, jersey, and blends that follow the line of the body are what you want. Fabric blends have evolved to make even luxury fibers like cashmere and alpaca stronger, to increase their wearability. Cashmere is often mixed with wools and synthetics to bring the price down and make it more durable. Microfiber coats with faux fur linings offer the same appeal of fluffy furs but without additional weight. Wool is water-repellent, and the crimped fibers are excellent at trapping air close to the body. The blending of cashmere or wool with synthetics like acrylic, polyester, nylon, Lycra®, or acetate provides ease of movement and breathability. For sportier styles like ski parkas, new synthetics wick away moisture. ●

A NO-FAT GUIDE TO COATS

Man-tailored topcoat

With a classic V-neck notch collar, this single- or double-breasted topper is cut like an expensive overcoat for men. The V-neck lapels and narrow tailored shape provide a lean look that lengthens your neck and streamlines the area from muffin top to tummy.

Ladylike coat

Fitted on top to the waist, it then flares to the hem. Often, there are slimming vertical princess seams from bust to hem, and trendier versions have sleeves that bell or puff out to the wrist. This style is terrific for bigger bottoms, hips, thighs, and rear and fat arms and tummy. You've seen it on Carla Bruni, Michelle Obama, Queen Elizabeth II—and in our No Fat look.

Sculpted coat

This one features dramatic contours—either a wide dolman shape or a curved cocoon shape. Some have deep armholes or raglan sleeves. Because it combines sharp architectural lines and volume, there is plenty of room for big boobs, rear, hips, and thighs and middle issues. Just FYI: You need height and fashion confidence to carry it off!

Retro coat

It looks vintage, but new fabrics and detailing put it in a contemporary context. It can be cut straight or A-lined, but it features looser cropped three-quarter sleeves, fancy collars, and decorative buttons. This coat skims past the middle, and all the attention on top is a great diversion for women with heavy thighs and legs. Just choose styles with buttons in matching tones if you are bosomy and shawl collars or notched lapels if you have a short neck.

Peacoat

This nautical-inspired style is a classic. That's good news. It comes in several coat lengths, from mid-thigh to knee grazing. Its body-skimming tailored shape is flattering. If you're really busty, however, a peacoat is not your best bet because your breasts will be smushed into one weird uni-boob. It's better for those who want to bulk up their tops to balance out wider bottom halves.

Empire coat

Mod inspired with raised waist, this coat totally hides a flabby midsection with a fashion-y look. Stick to solids and don't get sidetracked by fattening extras—such as plaid—that cancel the slimming effect.

Swing coat

Also called a trapeze style, this one starts out fitted at the shoulder then cuts loose to a triangle shape. Lots of middle-management opportunities here—as it's flattering on those with muffin top, Buddha belly, and a generous rear, plus, it shows off great legs.

Cape coat

Belted in front, deep and loose at the armholes, this style offers camouflage for back fat, arms, and big boobs and is super for larger sizes.

10 THINGS THAT MAKE YOU LOOK FAT IN A *Coat*

1. **Wearing a coat that pulls across the boobs,** hips, or rear, causing buttons, vents and pockets to gape.

2. **Choosing a short, waist-level jacket** that ends above the derriere and exposes all your lower body issues.

3. **Opting for the longest, fluffiest, puffiest down coat possible;** there are more slenderizing versions and proportions.

4. **Choosing the same style now that you wore when you were many pounds thinner.** The coat category in fashion has expanded and incorporated the same trends in design, details, color, and proportions that we now see in everyday clothes.

5. **Big, grid-like prints** like plaids or houndstooth that emphasize bulges rather than blurring them.

6. **Wearing a big, schlumpy coat** that doesn't show any womanly curves—there's a difference between menswear inspired and menswear. Even subtle shaping and tapered fit at the shoulder makes it more feminine.

7. **A light-colored coat versus a dark-colored coat.**

8. **Chasing the chill with a high stand-up collar** and textured muffler wound around and around that shortens the distance between neck and shoulders.

9. **Too many extras that increase size where you need it least,** like huge flap or patch pockets that exaggerate full hips, epaulettes that highlight broad shoulders, and wide lapels or big buttons that call attention to big boobs.

10. **Wearing belted jackets or belted sweaters under a belted coat.** Belted under belted is a huge "never" for everyone. This double belting squeezes and plumps you like those twisted-balloon figures at kids' birthday parties.

LAYER LIKE A PRO

Make "wide over narrow," "long over short" your seasonal mantra—this means a full cropped jacket over a high-waisted jersey dress, or a long tunic sweater over skinny jeans or a narrow pencil skirt, for example. You'd never want wide, full pants and a wide cropped jacket or a long sweater over a long, mid-calf skirt.

is the last. This is a major obstacle for women who try to wear chunky sweaters under fitted, tailored coats.

LET SOME AIR AND SKIN IN. Layers should float or skim around, not be so tightly stacked. You want to create the illusion of a body that can move.

LAYERING OVER A SKIRT IS THE SLIMMEST WAY TO GO because your legs on their own will always create a leaner vertical than your legs in pants, especially of you're wearing dark opaque tights and leg-hugging high-heel boots.

→ continued on page 196

> Here's the rule: No more than three layers at a time; four layers, if you count the coat.

Layering is in part a numbers game. If you layer a tank under a long-sleeve tee, under a big, cozy, thick sweater, under a cropped leather blazer and add slouchy pants, a big muffler, and a belted double-breasted military-style coat—and you are not one of the size 0 celebs in the tabloids—you will be visually adding 15 pounds to your frame. Here's the rule: No more than three layers at a time; four layers, if you count the coat.

KEEP THE LIGHTEST LAYER CLOSEST TO THE BODY and progressively build fabric weight out so the heaviest, thickest, bulkiest item

SWAP-OUTS:
CHICER WAYS TO HIDE FAT IN WINTER

Instead of →	Go for
A boxy stadium coat	A shaped-waist parka
A coat in plaid	A coat in a vibrant red
Head-to-toe black layers	Tonal grays, browns, or plums
Horizontal-striped sweaters	Vertical-ribbed sweaters
A long-cabled sweater coat	A hip-length grandpa cardigan
A thick muffler	A long, flat cashmere scarf
Wide lapels and collars	Narrow lapels or no collar
Wool mittens to match your coat	Leather-lined gloves

HIGH FAT *vs.* NO FAT

→ Let your coat do the work for you. The right one should shape you into an hourglass and give you a longer and leaner look. Chic it up with heeled boots that fit snug on the leg, and non-fat accessories.

....

HIGH FAT:
A light colored puffer coat packs on the pounds. The scarf, pom-pom hat, tucked in pants, and flat, patterned boots bulk you even more. A good look for kids.

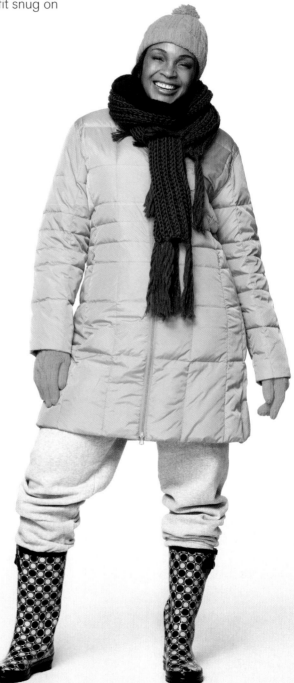

HOW FAST CAN YOU GIVE THESE AWAY?

HIGH FAT

× Flat, patterned boots

× Long, full skirts and big, cozy sweaters

× Pants tucked in boots

× Puffer with horizontal quilted puffs

× Thick, knit mufflers with fringe

NO FAT:
A black single-breasted coat that cinches your waist with an A-line bottom makes you look svelte, even in the cold. Oversized hats make your face look tiny.

YOU CAN'T HAVE TOO MANY OF THESE!

NO FAT

√ Buttons toned to jacket or coat

√ Cardigans worn open over sleeveless dresses

√ Hats that add volume—trappers, toques, full berets

√ Keeping all layers monochromatic—one color head to toe

√ Slim, stretchy black boots with a high heel

What a difference!

From frosty the snowman to a thin, cool, ice princess. Send that puffer packing!

STICK TO SOLIDS AND THE SAME COLOR FAMILY whenever possible for the leanest look. Mixing in texture is great, but plaids, checks, prints, and stripes mixed in with layers are fattening.

DON'T PILE ON A LOT OF BIG, BLACK, SHAPELESS PIECES— black does have a magical way of making every woman look thinner, but unless the pieces have some structure, they are not so magical and you can forget about looking Fit Not Fat.

KEEP NECKLINES FLATTERING. The worst offenders are double-breasted military styles with stand-up collars and chubby horizontally channeled puffer coats. Women with short necks and full bosoms look fat in these. Don't go larger to accommodate layering when deciding between two coat sizes. You'll end up looking bigger than you are. ●

A Layering Nightmare
If you layer a tank under a long-sleeve tee, under a big, cozy, thick sweater, under a cropped leather blazer and add slouchy pants, a big muffler, and a belted double-breasted military-style coat—and you are not one of the size 0 celebs in the tabloids—you will be visually adding 15 pounds to your frame.

BRILLIANT BRANDS
for coats

Banana Republic	**J. Crew**
Club Monaco	**Kohl's (Simply Vera)**
Diane von Furstenberg	**Liz Claiborne by Isaac Mizrahi**
DKNY	**Milly**
Gap	**Victoria's Secret**
H&M	

Thinner by Tonight!

INSTANT GRATIFICATION

Show some leg.
Wear skirts or dresses instead of pants, so the thinnest part of your body shows!

Shorten your coat-to-knee length.
It won't change the proportion of the coat but will add inches to your body to balance curves.

Opt for smooth knits rather than chunky, thick sweaters under coats. The warmth is in the fiber, not the thickness, of the sweater. Keep those thick-cabled sweaters for weekends at home in front of the fire—alone.

Add a vest, not a long-sleeved sweater for extra warmth if your arms are your big fat issue, and look for coats with roomy raglan, dolman, three-quarter, or bracelet sleeves.

Wear jackets or suits only under coats that can handle a structured layer—man-tailored topcoats, sculpted coats, peacoats, swing coats, and retro coats with deep armholes and fuller sleeves.

Don't close up from neck to chin if you can help it, but especially if you have a short neck and big bosom. Stick to V-neck coats with shawl or notch collars, and fill in necks for outdoors with a long, flat scarf looped, not wound, around so some neck is still visible.

How to loop: Fold a long scarf in half, holding an end in either hand. Center the scarf behind your neck and pull the loose open ends together and downward through the loop end. Adjust to fit.

Wear opaque black tights and matching slim knee-high boots to keep work-wear coats looking as slim as possible. Microfiber ones that have been water-proofed are terrific.

Wear a hat that adds volume to your head.
The popular fur or faux Russian hat, and fur or faux banded knit cap, expands the size of your head to balance bigger coat shapes so you don't look like a pinhead. Anything that squashes down your hair and makes your head smaller, like a knit cap, will make your body seem bigger. Those Elmer Fudd earflap hats are warm, but just realize when you're wearing it that it's not your most glam look.

WINTER SOLUTIONS

IF YOU'RE PETITE…

• WEAR COLOR ON THE OUTSIDE AND KEEP THE BASE NEUTRAL, DARK, AND TONED— like a tomato-red peacoat over a navy crew and dark blue jeans or a buttery yellow jacket over a tobacco suede skirt and matching sweater.

• INVEST IN BOOTS AND TIGHTS THAT WORK TOGETHER, and give your legs the slimmest line.

• LOOK FOR THREE-QUARTER COATS THAT WILL HOVER A FEW INCHES ABOVE YOUR KNEE, or in some cases these will reach your knee! It's more than okay if a little skirt shows.

• MAKE SURE THE COAT FITS SNUGLY AT THE SHOULDER, BUST, OR WAIST, even if it flares or billows below. You need to define your shape.

• LOOK FOR EMPIRE AND RAISED-WAIST STYLES that will stretch your torso and make you appear taller and slimmer.

• KEEP IT AS SIMPLE AS POSSIBLE. Solid colors with one major design detail high on the body, like a tie neck or contrasting collar, will help you look lean.

IF YOU'RE SIZE 14 & UP…

• WEAR COLOR ON THE INSIDE, AND PUT YOUR DARK NEUTRAL ON THE OUTSIDE—like a plum jersey dress and tights with a long, gray cardigan on top.

• ADD THE THICKEST, HEAVIEST LAYER ON TOP. A wide-sleeved A-line, trapeze, or empire coat fits easily over layers beneath.

• GO FOR TAILORED, UNBELTED COATS WITH STRAIGHT LINES OR VOLUME—swing coats and sculpted coats.

• LOOK FOR COLLARS WITH DRAMA. Fold-over funnels, cowls, and portrait necklines with a retro flair and fur (real or faux) collars bring the focus to your face.

• TRY CAPE COATS THAT TIE IN FRONT ONLY for subtle definition without an actual wraparound belt. These make layering easy and have a definite Aspen look.

Vows *for* Winter

☐ **I WILL NEVER** wear more than three layers of clothing at a time.

☐ **I WILL NOT** be seduced by trendy fattening pockets, belts, collars, and shoulder lines, no matter how hard designers try.

☐ **I WILL** skip all coats above my waist and below my knees.

☐ **I WILL** try on all my accessories with a new coat before removing the tags.

☐ **I WILL** finally give away my old, black, ankle-length puffer coat.

DON'T YOU DARE...

Wear a jazzy appliquéd sweater. Just because it's holiday time doesn't mean it's okay to go juvenile. Holiday themes featuring reindeer prints, Christmas trees, gift boxes decorated with pom-poms, appliqués, fringe, and big ball buttons will add width or attention to the wrong spots. If you want to go festive, wear a red or green sweater with a neutral bottom to anchor the festivity!

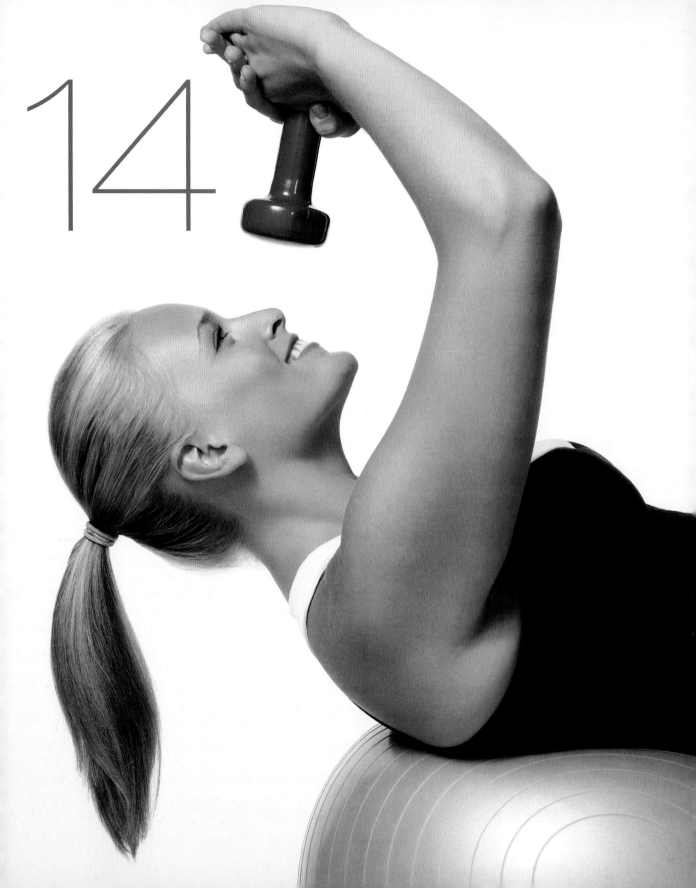

14

Workout Wear

YOU THINK YOU LOOK FAT IF . . .

Your sports bra gives you a uni-boob . . . You wonder who that out-of-shape person is when you see your reflection in the wall-to-wall mirrors at the gym . . . You wear a fanny pack . . . Your workout gear is an advertisement for your college/high school/sports team . . . The thought of wriggling into a stretchy spandex top or bottom is enough reason not to work out at all . . . You can't remember the last time you bought sneakers.

→Thinking about what to wear when you work out may sound like a big, fat waste of time and the last thing you want to do. Most of us are just so happy that we are even going to exercise that we tend not to care what we wear. We throw on any old pair of baggy sweatpants with bleach spots, paint splats, or coffee stains and then add an oversized T–shirt to this high-fat mix. The T–shirt is probably a goodie-bag giveaway with a company logo on it, or that of a vacation place, or our favorite college, or a meant-to-be-funny saying. I am by no means suggesting that you get all dolled up for the gym or a spin class. (A full face of makeup when you're working out looks ridiculous, but a little tinted moisturizer will give you a good glow!)

Still, you don't want to look or feel fat when you're exercising because it's so incredibly self-defeating. With walls of mirrors surrounding you, you're forced to watch yourself as you sweat it out. You'll be so much more inspired if that image staring back at you is wearing something that supports and complements your figure rather than something that hides it or displays it Hooters-style. When you look at your reflection, you don't ever want to think, *Why should I bother?*

Looking Fit Not Fat in your workout wear is not just about vanity; it's about your motivation. Tracy Anderson, fitness trainer to Gwyneth Paltrow and Madonna, is all about getting the most from your time investment. "If you like what you're wearing and you're comfortable in it, then you're going to be totally focused on your performance," she says. In other words, if you're not bashing yourself for looking fat, your mind can focus on your form. And you won't be so mortified about how you look that you can't concentrate on the task at hand when you run into someone from work. It happens to all of us. And, consider the possibility that you could meet your soul mate while waiting for the elliptical. As the world now knows, Jessica Seinfeld met her husband at the Reebok Sports Club on Manhattan's Upper West Side. I don't know what she was wearing at the time, but having been a member there, I will bet you a Lululemon tank top that it wasn't a pair of elastic waistband sweats and size XXL tee! If rethinking your workout wear is tough for you, put it on your WIMP (When I'm Mentally Prepared) list. ●

for Workouts

→ IF YOU HAVEN'T BOUGHT NEW exercise clothes since aerobicizing with Jane Fonda in a unitard (don't laugh; I just threw mine out!), your heart-rate monitor will rev up when you see the brands, styles, quality, and fabrics you could be wearing. If you don't care one whit about style, you still need to know about the state-of-the-art wicking fabrics that keep you dry as you sweat, even if your workout is Sweatin' to the Oldies (with Richard Simmons). Trust me on this. They're sensual, too,

category is booming, as workout clothes have become fashion.

"My big dream for the Adidas collaboration is to give women performance garments that they look great in but not sacrifice design," fashion "It girl" Stella McCartney told *Women's Wear Daily*. Her line for Adidas is as hip as her namesake collection, with warm-up jackets in chic metallics, running pants in electric blue and sea green, and yoga gear in fleshy nudes and pale pinks. Yohji Yamamoto, Christy Turlington,

That there are chains of chic boutiques that sell nothing but yoga and running clothes tells you that the activewear category is booming, as workout clothes have become fashion.

much sexier to wear than bulky cottons. Whether or not you actually do yoga or run, go online or take a field trip to one of the Lululemon stores in the United States (there are sixty-five at press time) to learn what's current in workout gear, such as reflective clothing so that you can run after dark, or hidden pockets so you can be hands-free. That there are chains of chic boutiques that sell nothing but yoga and running clothes tells you that the activewear

and Alexander McQueen are a few more big names designing athletic wear in fashion colors way beyond black or navy. Lululemon and Lucy use bright pink, deep purple, and lime green in their collections. As the ad from the hip Lucy brand declares, "We're on a divine mission to free women from the servitude of insidious workout fashion." You can just hear women everywhere saying, amen!

With so many fun, flattering, and

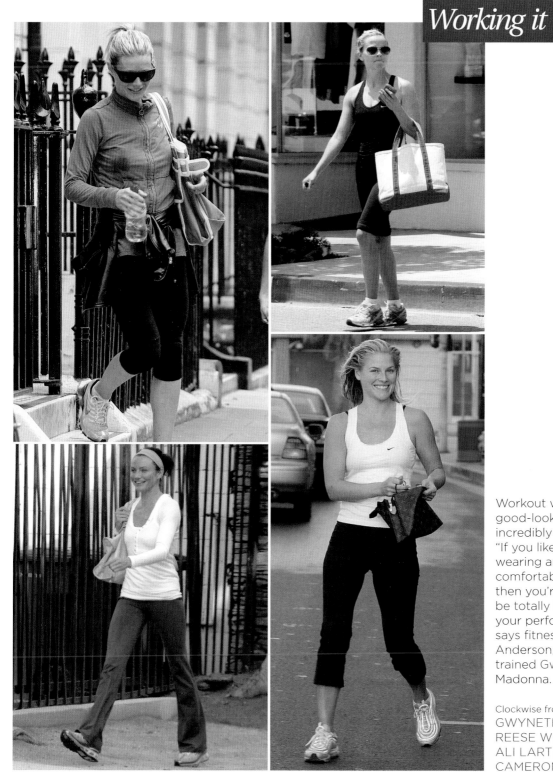

Workout wear this good-looking is incredibly motivating. "If you like what you're wearing and you're comfortable in it, then you're going to be totally focused on your performance," says fitness guru Tracy Anderson, who has trained Gwyneth and Madonna.

Clockwise from top left: GWYNETH PALTROW, REESE WITHERSPOON, ALI LARTER, CAMERON DIAZ

ultra-comfy options in halter tops, tanks, yoga pants, and hoodies, you might be tempted to substi-

Workout gear on city streets in downtown Chicago or New York's Madison Avenue looks as undressed as your feet in a pair of flip-flops.

tute activewear for street wear—for running errands, brunching, shopping in the mall—and spend the day in yoga pants and hoodie. Don't, unless you live a charmed, laid-back lifestyle near the beach. While it's appropriate in Miami, Malibu, Santa Monica, all of Southern California, and Hawaii, workout gear on city streets in downtown Chicago or New York's Madison Avenue looks as undressed as your feet in a pair of flip-flops. Even if it is super-cute and hot pink from Juicy! I know I'm going to regret saying this, but a Juicy sweatsuit looks "trying-too-hard" on a body over the age of thirty-five—even at the airport.

For long flights, a pair of comfy pants with stretch or a dress with a pair of leggings underneath is so much chicer than walking around in workout wear when everyone knows that *1)* you did have time to change clothes, and *2)* you are not going to be working out in flight.

Before we get to what to wear, let's talk one more second about what not to wear at the gym. Some women flash their six-pack abs in midriff tops with yoga pants rolled down dangerously low. Is this kind of aggressive dressing really necessary? It's so Mean Girls. Memo to all exhibitionists: Have a little compassion for the women you see around you. We don't have to be so competitive with one another. We're all trying to get fit! ●

YOUR NO-FAT GYM LOOK

Invest in at least two of these ultra-flattering, fashion-forward workout outfits so you always have a clean one to put on.

Whatever your sport, there's a cool new crop of clothes specifically designed to make you excel, and look Fit Not Fat while you're at it. Invest in at least two of these ultra-flattering, fashion-forward workout outfits so you always have a clean one to put on. All your pieces should be in high-tech fabrics that wick sweat away from your body and let you move around comfortably, fitting you like a not-too-tight second skin.

"I'm a fan of fitted shapes—you want to see what you look like," says Vicky McGarry, who styled her share of workout shoots as fashion director of *Women's Health* magazine. If you're still wearing shapeless cotton clothing, you're going to look dated and frumpy. The key pieces:

YOGA PANTS. Even if your exercise routine doesn't require a yoga-body look, invest in yoga pants. They work as general all-around workout pants, depending on the length. If you're a yoga practioner, you'll find that the styles that flare at the bottom are universally flattering. If you're spinning, the pants should hit somewhere between → *continued on page 208*

→ *continued on page 208*

10 THINGS THAT MAKE YOU LOOK FAT IN *Workout Wear*

1. **Fanny packs.** Instead, choose a pant with hidden pockets to hold your credit card and keys for hands-free walking. As convenient as fanny packs are, we tend not to see how bulky and unflattering they can be. Check out your side view in the mirror.

2. **Short, stretchy, black bike shorts that hit you mid-thigh.**

3. **Old-school gym and running shorts.**

4. **A sweaty white T–shirt** with a white sports bra underneath.

5. **Track pants with zippered pockets up and down the legs.**

6. **Running shorts that flash the world your thighs.**

7. **A sports bra worn as a top.**

8. **Pants in a loud color—** stick to dark on the bottom.

9. **Two sports bras at the same time for support.**

10. **Your sweatshirt tied around your waist.** This has the same effect as a fanny pack. Why add more to your middle?

HIGH FAT *vs.* NO FAT

→ Don't throw on any old thing when you go to exercise. If you look great, you'll be more motivated to hang in there. Once you invest in workout clothes that flatter your shape, you'll never want to take them off!

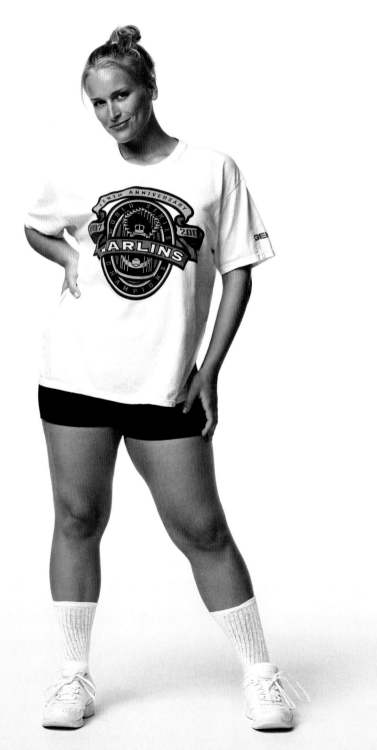

HIGH FAT:
A supersized tee and short shorts will supersize you. White sneakers and tube socks is the equivalent of ice cream mixed with pieces of cookie dough.

HOW FAST CAN YOU GIVE THESE AWAY?

HIGH FAT

× Bulky sweatshirts

× Oversized T–shirts

× Running shorts

× Spandex bike shorts

× Sweatpants with letters on the seat

× White sneakers with tube socks

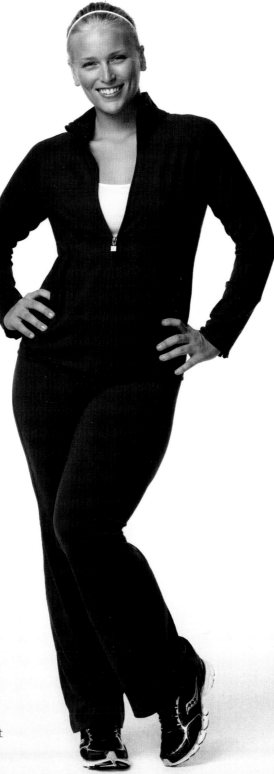

What a difference!

The figure-enhancing No Fat outfit keeps your secrets under cover while the High Fat not only blabs, but exaggerates.

NO FAT:
A long dark line, down to the sneakers, creates a slimming vertical from simple stretch pieces that skim the body without screaming for attention.

YOU CAN'T HAVE TOO MANY OF THESE!

NO FAT

√ Sleek, fitted sweat jackets

√ Burnout long-sleeve tees for layering

√ Gray or black sports bras

√ Stretchy, solid empire-waist shimmel or tank tops

√ Tone-on-tone prints

√ Yoga pants

Thinner by Tonight!

INSTANT GRATIFICATION

Swap your sweat-stained white T–shirt for a tank top in a rich jewel tone.

Throw on a tissue-thin long-sleeved T-shirt over your tank top instead of an oversized sweatshirt.

Tie your hair back with a black, no-tangle elastic band. Throw out those scrunchies!

Carry a cute tote bag to hold your gym gear instead of a bulky duffel.

Slip on cropped black yoga pants—the most universally flattering workout bottoms.

Swap your white jog bra for a sports bra in black or a color.

Wear a thong to the gym. VPL underneath form-fitting workout pants is an eyesore. Plus, you will feel sexier.

Unzip your hoodie and show some cleavage.

Wear a skinny headband to keep back your bangs; not a head scarf.

---

the knee and the calf, as any longer and they'll interfere with the pedals of the bike. For spinning, you might also try pants that fit tight (rather than flare) on the leg. Whatever length, you want to see some skin (the operative word being *some*), even if it's just the ankles. Choose the length most comfortable for you in the forgiving shades of black, navy, brown, or gray.

"Across the board, black bottoms look good on everyone," say Vicky. "Beware low-cut pants that are short waisted—you'll get muffin top. Lululemon has a roll-top waistband that can extend up to cover your belly." Roll-top yoga pants let you decide how low you want to go at the waist.

A SHIMMEL TOP. You'll feel like you have proper coverage in these long, full tank tops. If you're an A–C cup, choose a shimmel top with a shelf bra or built-in bra. The top can be a scoop neck, halter top, racerback, or empire waist. Empire is flattering for those looking to hide a serious tummy. If you have a more ample bust, you may want the support of a sports bra under a stretchy nylon T-shirt. "Always opt for the most high-tech fabric," Vicky says, and she recommends the Nike tees made of Dri-FIT technology to keep you cool and dry. So that you don't get stuck in an all-black rut, choose a pretty color on top. "Blues and pinks always look good and are universally appealing in women's apparel," says Vicky. "Orange is going to change with fashion, and so is green." Be wary of prints, unless they're subtle tone on tone; they'll do nothing but pack on the pounds. Those old, holey cotton T–shirts? They make great rags.

A LAYERING SHIRT OR SWEAT JACKET. Over your tank top, you want to layer either a lightweight long-sleeved T–shirt or a fitted sweat jacket. "I think it's really important to have layers," says trainer Tracy Anderson. "A lot of microfibers can be too tight, so I wear a lot of burnout tees that are perfect for layering." Burnout fabric, which feels like it's been washed a thousand times, is featherweight soft and light. Choose these super-

Make sure your jacket is fitted, flirty, and feminine.

fine cottons and you'll never look bulky. When you start getting hot, you can peel off the layers. If you live in a cold climate, you might layer a sweat jacket instead of a long-sleeve tee. Make sure your jacket is

fitted, flirty, and feminine in soft fabrics like nylon, Lycra[®], lightweight cotton, or jersey. The fit should delicately drape your body, creating a nice line, but it should never be so tight so as to bunch up (and make you look fat).

A SPORTS BRA. Buy a non-white sports bra, maybe one in gray, black, or a color. If you want to keep your bra on the DL, buy nude. "Traditionally women wear white, but a white bra has a tendency to show through your clothes, especially after you have perspired," says Liz Smith, director of retail services at Wacoal America. If you're going to flash the public your underwear, then it might as well be pretty. Make sure that the fit is perfect to avoid irritation and jiggle. "Compression and encapsulation are the two key terms to understand when it comes to sports bras," says Smith. "The right sports bra should lift and support your breast tissue, not just smash and flatten your bust. You shouldn't have to sacrifice a nice shape and silhouette while working out. You need to keep the girls supported and in place or eventually they'll just start heading south." You want to avoid the uni-boob, created when both breasts are pushed together so tight that they become one large horizontal breast. Let's just say it does the opposite of make you look thin.

SNEAKERS. "Wear black or silver shoes to make your feet look smaller," says Vicky. "We've evolved from white sneakers. You'll look like a novice if you're wearing bright white."

Be wary of prints, unless they're subtle tone on tone; they'll do nothing but pack on the pounds. Those old, holey cotton T–shirts? They make great rags.

SOCKS. Regardless of what pant length you choose, letting old-fashioned cotton socks that cover your ankle and ride up to an un-flattering place on your leg will ruin your no fat workout look. Instead of bulky tube socks, wear Ped-like cotton socks (such as Spanx Sport-Ease! athletic low-rise socks; even Madonna is a fan) that barely peek out of your sneakers. ●

BRILLIANT BUYS

WORKOUT WEAR

TOPS

LuLulemon Define Jacket, $99; lululemon.com.

Champion Seamless Empire Long Top, style 2936, $36; championusa.com. Updated fabrication.

New Balance Versatility Cami, 34A/32 B to 40DD, style WBT8301, $50; newbalance.com.

BOTTOMS

LuLulemon Groove Pant, $98; lululemon.com.

Marika Miracles Miraculous Butt Booster Capri with Tummy Control, style MM5095, $45; marika.com.

Marika Miracles Miraculous Thigh Slenderizer Pant with Tummy Control, style MM5096, $48; marika.com.

Nike Women Nike Pacer Women's Running Skirt, style 364046 in black or reflective silver, $45; nikewomen.com.

Nike Women Dri-Fit Be Strong Regular Pant, style 339532-010, $40; nikewomen.com.

Nike Women Dri-Fit Be Bold Slim Capri, style 354566-010, $50; nikewomen.com.

Teez-Her The Skinny Capri, style 229TP793, $36; Dillard's, Von Mauer.

SOCKS

Spanx Sportease! Advanced Athletic Low-Rise Socks, $10; spanx.com.

SPORTS BRAS

Bendon Sport Max Out High Impact Underwire Bra, 34B–40DD, $55; barenecessities.com.

Le Mystere Energie Sports Bra, style 320, 32–40 B–G, $64; Nordstrom, barenecessities.com.

Lululemon Ta Ta Tamer, style LW2267S, 32B–38DD, in five colors, $58; lululemon.com. It's been said to "fit like armor"!

Natori Sport Underwire Bra, 32B–40DDD, style 7234439, $48; Intimacy, bareneccessesties.com.

Wacoal Sport Underwire Sports Bra, style 855170, 32–40C, D, DDD, $62; Nordstrom, barenecessities.com.

BEST BRANDS

Adidas by Stella McCartney; adidas.com.

Athletica pants and tops; athletica.net.

Lucy.com pants and tops; lucy.com.

Lululemon pants and tops; lululemon.com.

Marika Miracles shape enhancing activewear; marika.com.

Nikewomen clothing and shoes. nikewomen.com.

Nuala by Puma; puma.com.

Yohji Yamamoto for Adidas; y-3store.adidas.com.

Vows *for* Workout Wear

☐ **I WILL NOT** put on a sports bra that gives me a uni-boob.

☐ **I WILL NEVER** work out in bike shorts.

☐ **I WILL NEVER** wear a top that flaunts my belly button.

☐ **I WILL NOT** wear a fanny pack while jogging.

☐ **I WILL NEVER** wear socks that go above my ankle.

☐ **I WILL NOT** wear scrunchies in the gym.

☐ **I WILL NOT** wear a ratty old T–shirt and sweatpants.

☐ **I WILL NOT** wear pants with lettering across my butt.

DON'T YOU DARE . . .

Justify an excessive amount of calories because you've worked out. Rather than keep a food diary in your handbag, a new way to keep track of your daily calories is to download the app "Lose It" at the Apple iTunes store. It calculates your daily calories for you.

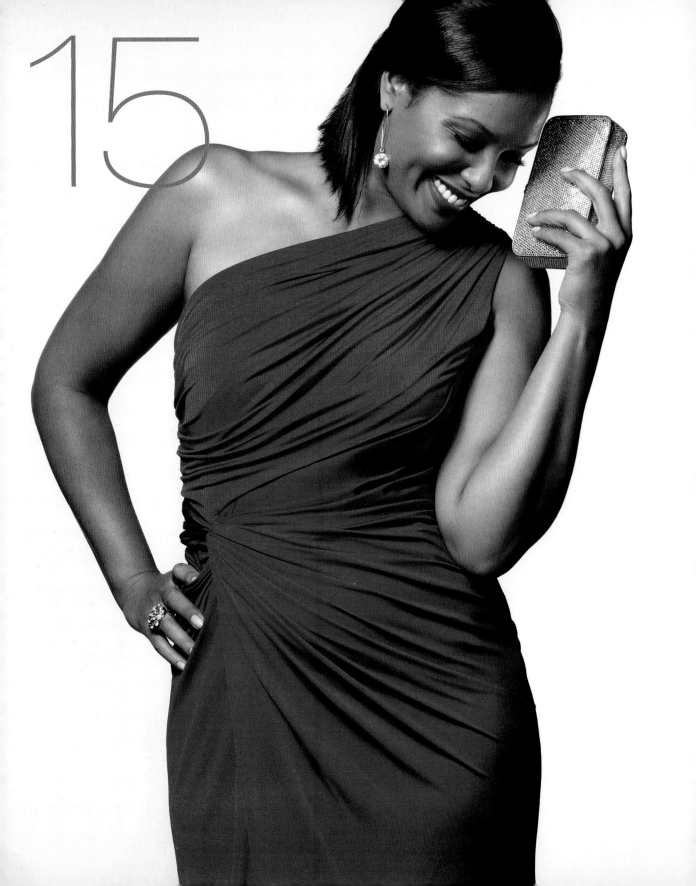

15

Evening

YOU THINK YOU LOOK FAT IF...
You turn down invitations to events because you don't have anything to wear . . . You're layering not one but two body-shapers just to zip up . . . Your fallback is an old tuxedo . . . You spent the evening holding your breath because your dress must have shrunk since the last time you wore it . . . You borrow your husband's jacket, saying you're cold when you're not.

→ Every woman I know loves watching the arrivals at the Oscars more than watching the show itself. You couldn't ask for a better lesson in high-fat/no-fat glamour. The no-fat award in 2009 went to Kate Winslet. Not only did she win the Oscar, but she won the night in a one-shoulder, waist-defining, gray satin YSL dress that flattered her curvy shape without hiding it. The high-fat award in 2009 went to Jessica Biel. Her ivory-satin Prada origami-folded strapless, with excess draping, proved that just because it's designer, expensive, and off-the-runway fashion doesn't mean it does great things for a body, even a stunning body like hers.

Aside from our red carpet fascination, we live in a culture that requires most women to get really dressed up in formal black tie or even semi-dressy attire rather infrequently. Gone are the days when you would get all decked out in hats with netting, opera-length gloves, stoles, or boas just to go out to dinner on a Saturday night like our mothers did. But even if you're not on the charity circuit, chances are you still have at least a few occasions a year—business events, weddings, anniversaries, and bar and bat mitzvahs—that call for a major all-out effort.

For decades, the fallback plan for women of style has been the LBD (little black dress). With good reason. It is the no-fat choice that can make you look thinner, taller, more confident, and chic . . . but not every black dress works. Some LBDs are frumpy, baggy, and fattening as a muumuu. We're talking about baby-dolls, bubble dresses, and dowdy mid-calf slipdresses that don't flatter anyone. If you are not the LBD type, you should really try to be. All you have to do is find one, just one, that makes you look Fit Not Fat, and you're home free.

Has your approach to fancy dressing been "Oh, I'll just put on a pair of black pants and a dressy top and be done with it"? C'mon, fess up! Have you ever uttered those words? Sure you have. Most of us have muttered those words and even more than once. Black pants with a dressy top or jacket is a popular formula that's inherently trickier than it seems. It's hard to find that perfect top! Not to mention stressful and time-consuming. Many a well-meaning woman has tried . . . she ends up in a bulge-making sheer or sequin or ill-fitting top that has the look of an outfit thrown together at the last minute. Take a good look around the room next time you're at a party and you'll see what I mean. ●

YOUR DRESS-THINNER STRATEGY
for Evening

→ SOME WOMEN WOULD RATHER have laser hair removal than shop for something to wear to a black-tie affair! They probably feel that the pressure is on and that they need to reinvent themselves for the occasion. But I'm here to tell you that there is no need to change your personal style or body-flattering strategy . . . just follow the same plan in dressier fabrics with fancier accessories. If your "go to" day look is an empire-waist dress with a V neckline and soft sleeves, it might be your best bet for evening, too. If tunics work for you, look for glitzier versions and wear them over slim pants with metallic or jeweled heels after six. You'll look St. Tropez chic.

Before we figure out your best no-fat look for evening, let's decipher the dress codes. "Black tie" today means either short or long and everything in between, with short, currently, having the edge over long. Women who skirt the issue by wearing an asymmetrical handkerchief hem, which is both short and long, sometimes end up looking dowdy. "Black tie optional" translates into a short dressy dress. "Formal attire" means a long dress or skirt. "Creative black tie" means short, or call your host for further explanation! Where dress is not indicated on the invite, you're left to

crack the code on your own. Where you live might help you to determine how dressy to get, but for an evening event in a big city—a class reunion, a holiday cocktail party, a gallery opening—you will look Fit Not Fat in a knee-skimming dress with an embellished coat or cardigan. At this fashion moment, the

> I'm here to tell you that there is no need to change your personal style or body-flattering strategy . . . just follow the same plan in dressier fabrics with fancier accessories.

dressy evening skirt suit often worn by mothers-of-the-bride in a heavy fabric is passé. A sexy, fitted pantsuit can look modern; a boxy workaday pantsuit or skirt suit does not, even if you have jazzed it up with a sexy camisole underneath—it's still a boxy suit. For a cocktail party after work, if you're already wearing a sleeveless LBD or a black pencil skirt, you can ramp up your look and appear more festive by merely adding a sequin cardigan, higher heels,

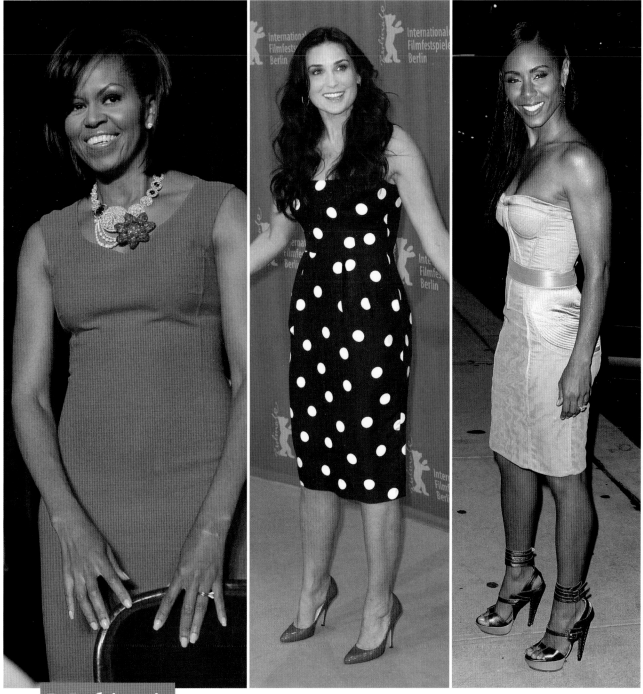

Working it

Girls' night out: Looking glam, without wearing all-black.
MICHELLE OBAMA, DEMI MOORE, JADA PINKETT SMITH

sparkly earrings, and a metallic clutch. And yes, you can add all—or some—of the above.

The event should dictate just how much skin to show. If it's a big nighttime glamorama event like a fund-raiser or a wedding, you can go a little more dramatic, showing cleavage at the neckline or back.

Here's a general rule I've learned about no-fat evening dressing: If the cut is simple and clean, you may be able to afford the "calories" of a wow fabric, shiny texture, or flashy color.

For work-related parties, forgo showing excess skin and maintain a sense of professionalism; women who don't risk looking slutty. If the party involves dancing, be sure you can move in your outfit and stand in your heels. Having to kick your shoes off at a glam affair is never a good idea . . . you lose height and gain weight.

Here's a general rule I've learned about no-fat evening dressing: If the cut is simple and clean, you may be able to afford the "calories" of a

wow fabric, shiny texture, or flashy color. The opposite, however, is not true. Wear a cut that's complicated and gimmicky and you could look high fat, even in a simple cotton or basic black. If you combine a tricky shape with a high-caloric fabric, you're cooking up a fattening recipe for disaster, the kind that often lands on the "What Was She Thinking?" sections of the celebrity tabloids.

Example of this theory: Because I'm vertically challenged, I look best in tailored-to-the-body dresses without a lot of volume and frou-

frou. Although I'd love to wear a big tulle ball gown (à la Sarah Jessica Parker at the Oscars 2009), it would look silly on me, as if I were auditioning to be a Disney princess at the Magic Kingdom. One of my favorite LBDs is a simple black sheath with a crew neckline and three-quarter sleeves—but it's all sequins—from Tory Burch. It works because the cut is as simple as the fabrication is flashy. It's my best no-fat look for evening. You can never go wrong with a dress like that. ●

SWAP-OUTS:
SWITCH FROM HIGH-FAT TO NO-FAT EVENING LOOKS

Instead of	→	Go for
Hair pinned up		Hair down with volume
A pouffy ball gown		A draped-front halter gown
A shiny lamé dress		A matte jersey dress
A slit to the thigh		A knee-length dress
A strapless mini		A strapless knee length sheath
A tuxedo look		A fitted pantsuit
Your old black LBD		A one-shoulder sheath

A NO-FAT GUIDE TO EVENING WEAR

Medium or small busted. Try strapless, one-shoulder, or halter styles. Strapless dresses are always top sellers because they showcase shoulders (which most women feel comfortable showing, because their shoulders still look good) and toned arms while leaving the rest to the imagination. The newer neckline, however, is the one-shoulder. That said, there are also new versions of strapless that do offer lift, camouflage, and coverage for body problems in both knee length and long versions.

Strapless dresses in empire-waist styles flow gently under the bust and when enhanced with draped or tiered fabric make good choices for flabby middles and Buddha bellies. Renee Zellweger's lemon-yellow strapless vintage dress she wore at the 2001 Oscars was a huge influence that kicked off this trend. More structured strapless styles with a defined waist and fuller A-line skirts disguise full thighs and a derriere; just choose thicker fabrics that won't cling to your skin.

For women with sun-damaged chests who want to wear the LBD strapless, some designers have addressed the issue by adding a sheer-illusion black-chiffon sleeveless part that continues to the neck like a sleeveless shell.

Big busted, flappy-armed, or broad shouldered. Strapless can be tricky. Abby Z., a stylist, designer, and retailer for larger sizes, says that you should never even think of wearing a strapless black dress the way it is in the store if you're a larger size. "You want to make one major adjustment, especially if your boobs are D or bigger. Buy black taffeta fabric, and have your tailor make one-inch straps to hide your bra straps under it. The taffeta straps will give any black strapless dress a lift. If you have heavy breasts plus back fat and belly fat, you will look slimmer in another style." This tip about hiding your bra straps happens to be one of my favorite tips because it allows bigger-busted women to go "strapless" with ease.

Shrugs and beaded cardigans can turn bare dresses you may have passed up into very appealing and wearable options. Yes, you can wear sleeveless if you don't ever take the cover-up off, so a new world of dresses opens up to you when you're shopping. Choose dress/jacket combos and dress/coat combos that are the newest twist on the twinset idea.

Hiding a tummy, back fat, and arms. Try a dressy jacket in a luxury fabric like velvet. There are lots of little cropped beaded and sequined sweaters on the racks just for this purpose. Some department stores even place them in accessories, on the ground floor.

Camouflaging muffin tops and flappy arms. Wear softer draped blouses and tops with ruffles, draped necklines, and graceful voluminous sleeves on top of slim, tailored black pants and skirts.

Counteracting muffin tops, a flabby middle, or a belly. Look for fabrics that are generously ruched, draped, or gathered to blur bulges. Even fitted, structured shapes like sheath dresses incorporate these features now. (See our No Fat look, page 221.)

Downplaying a hefty bosom. Emphasize the lower body in a pencil skirt in metallic leather or sequins worn with a simple V-neck sweater or T-shirt and jewel-studded cuffs. Don't be afraid to mix day and evening pieces creatively—remember Sharon Stone's famous black Gap T-shirt worn with a Valentino skirt. One-shoulder dresses are a great sexy alternative to cleavage-revealing looks. They actually cover the chest but show your curves—the only thing you need is an amazing strapless bra.

10 THINGS THAT MAKE YOU LOOK FAT IN *Evening Wear*

1. **Mid-calf skirt lengths.** Either knee-length or all-the-way-down formal. Anything else looks dowdy.

2. **Teen-targeted minis.** Not going thigh-high is a given if you're over thirty and/or have chunky legs.

3. **Droopy boobs unsupported under evening dresses.** Get 'em up with a well-fitted strapless bra.

4. **Too much cleavage.** Showing excessive amounts of breast with a maximum volume push-up bra or skimpy-top dress is a no-go. Unless you are in a Shakespeare play.

5. **Pouf and fluff.** Even if the goal is to let your legs star, a band of marabou feathers, big cha-cha ruffles, or puffy ballooning at the hem adds pounds to your lower body.

6. **Breaking the body up at the waist.** If the middle is your danger zone, skip the complications of piece-y tops and bottoms, belts, and jackets and go the dress route. This is doubly true if you are five-foot-four or under. An empire, raised waistline, one-shoulder column style with no defined break at the middle will neatly glide over belly and muffin top issues.

7. **Big, splashy prints.** Solids truly do work best for evening—and the range of color options is so dazzling, why risk making your butt look like it was upholstered? And no matter how tempting or trendy the designer name, stay away from big, chintzy cabbage roses, rainbow stripes, and complicated pictorial scenes that would make amazing wallpaper.

8. **Sugary debutante dresses.** Anything remotely resembling the Sugarplum Fairy or what you wore to your first wedding or christening is out. Frothy white dresses, big bows or sashes, Victorian looks, and puffy sleeves are super-fattening.

9. **Wearing a boxy tux.** If you go this route, choose a sexy style that is so fitted to your curves it couldn't possibly be mistaken for menswear.

10. **Excessive shine.** Take the shiny metallics down a notch to a muted sheen or use them strategically. Head-to-toe gold or silver sequins—or even neckline to knees—is hard for models to pull off. Just a flash of shine at the neckline or in small doses—a shrug or cardigan, a jeweled clutch, or gold-threaded silk or brocade—is tasteful not tacky and low-calorie.

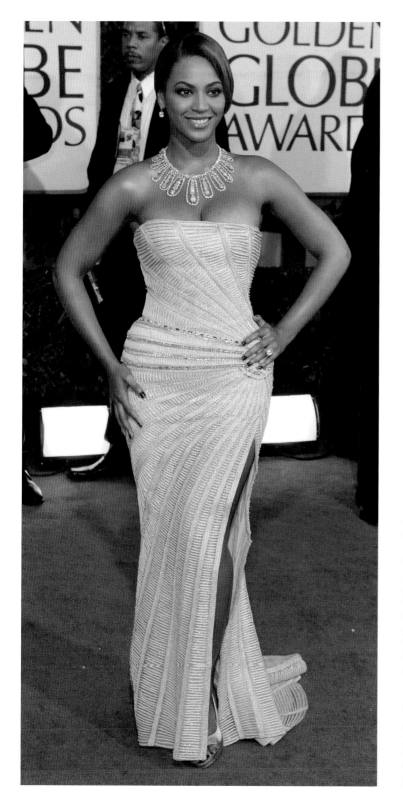

Just FYI: A dress with high-fat elements—light in color, metallic threads, thigh-high slit—can still look absolutely smashing if you possess the height, the bod, and the swagger to pull it off with confidence. Like BEYONCÉ does here.

To Look Thinner in Photos

Turn almost sideways and put one foot in front, toe pointed toward the camera. Keep your weight on your back leg, and bend the arm facing the camera at the elbow, and tighten by pressing your hand into your hip or waist (whichever you want to slim more) and smile over the photographer's head, pulling chin forward a bit from the neck—think "swan neck"—to eliminate any sag beneath. Practice; you'll get the hang of it. Never let anyone shoot you if she or he is crouching below—it adds ten pounds.

HIGH FAT *vs.* NO FAT

→ It's counterintuitive, for sure, but when
you need to ramp up for a glam night on
the town, have the confidence to practice
some restraint. Piling on layers of fattening
elements—color, shine, volume—is triple-
decker-sandwich caloric, not to mention
a little goofy-looking.

....

HIGH FAT:
Tulle skirt = big butt.
Strapless = back fat.
Turquoise sequins =
all eyes on your backside.
Oversized earrings +
upswept hair + too-mini
+ high heels = you haven't
got a chance in this outfit!

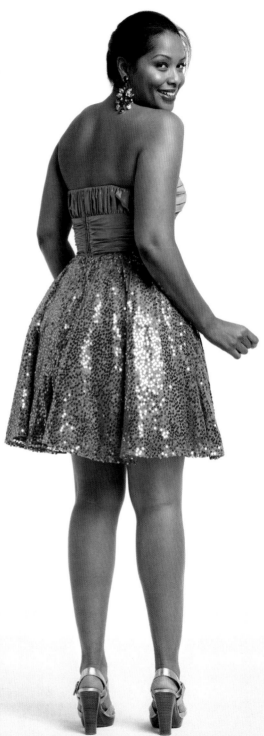

HOW FAST CAN YOU GIVE THESE AWAY?

HIGH FAT

× Clunky heels

× Bustier dresses

× Mid-calf dresses

× Pouffy dresses, skirts

× Sequin tube tops and boxy
  beaded shells

× Shapeless, long black skirts
  and dinner jackets

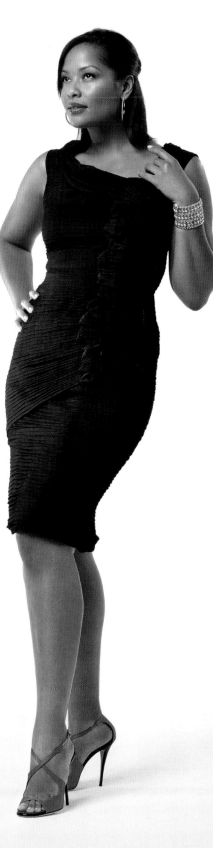

What a difference!

You'll never look slimmer than in a LBD. Leave vibrant sequin poufs on the rack for teen queens.

NO FAT:
There's a reason we keep coming back to a black dress. This hot little number displays a long ruffle that draws the eye down to a sizzling shoe. A winner!

YOU CAN'T HAVE TOO MANY OF THESE!

NO FAT

√ Broad V, scoopneck, neck-revealing LBDs

√ Halter dresses with draped fronts

√ One-shoulder or off-the-shoulder solid-colored jewel-tone dresses

√ Sexy pantsuits with nipped-waist jackets and lean pants

√ Strategic ruching across the midsection

√ Wide, low, square-neck sheaths with wide straps or sleeves

Thinner by Tonight!

INSTANT GRATIFICATION

Wear a silky slip as a liner under dresses so the dress fabric flows instead of sticking to your skin and body contours, says stylist Abby Z. Choose a slip that doubles as a body smoother. (See Brilliant Buys, page 224.)

Load up on jewels.
Long necklaces can help stretch a short neck and bring focus front and center, away from muffins, hips, and belly. Shorter mid-chest bibs, chunky pendants, or big chandeliers can move the eye from boobs to your face and keep them there. Sparkly cuffs, stacks of bangles, and cocktail rings can call attention to wrists instead of flabby upper arms.

Get a lift.
A great bra and body-shaper are essentials. In fact, splurge on the best underpinnings and give any dress a better shot at looking like it cost a million.

Wear a wide V neckline.
It will break up the heaviness of a full, wide chest. This can take a variety of formats: a V-neck velvet or silk jacket, a V-neck sheath or raised-waist dress, a ruffled or appliquéd cardigan with opened extra buttons to form a V, or a V-neck taffeta-wrap dress.

Pump up the hair.
Skip the fancy up-dos and hair accessories. Maxing out volume with a body-building shampoo, styling products, and a fresh blow-out makes the most of your hair. Hair that is collarbone length or longer will balance a fuller body.

Wear straight heels
in slingback or d'Orsay style or a tapered-toe pump to elongate your legs. Best for day dress-up are nudes to match your leg's skin tone and even two inches of heel helps.

Throw on a dressy coat.
Worn open, an evening coat will pare down the sides of your body so the center appears slimmer. Another reason to put a dress-coat duo on your to-buy list instead of a skirt suit.

Self-tan.
I cannot stress the confidence this little tint of color adds when you're baring a lot of skin. All those brown spots, veins, and discolorations meld together in a uniform color with a hint of glow.

Beat bloat.
Lie on the floor and elevate your feet against a wall for fifteen minutes to drain fluid that may have accumulated in your ankles. Sip hot water and lemon or fennel tea to dispel gas. Skip the salt the day before—that includes salt in mustard, ketchup, sushi, soups, soda, and Twizzlers!

EVENING SOLUTIONS

IF YOU'RE PETITE...

• LOOK FOR ONE-SHOULDER STYLES AND EMPIRES with one big detail, like a tie at the shoulder or a pleated bodice.

• LET RUCHING BLUR BULGES that even matte black can't hide effectively.

• WEAR KNEE-LENGTH DRESSES rather than long, even to black tie. You need the legginess for length and to create a slim line. It's okay, really.

• USE SHRUGS (mini cardigans) to help camouflage arms and back fat rather than opt for looser dress styles that can look baggy and shapeless on a small frame.

• SKYSCRAPER HEELS WILL GIVE YOU A LIFT but they can look out of proportion, and call attention to themselves if you're tottering because they kill.

• TOO POINTY A TOE ON A PETITE CAN LOOK LIKE WITCH SHOES. Wear a more conservative shoe, and you won't have to dance barefoot.

IF YOU'RE SIZE 14 & UP...

• TRY OFF-THE-SHOULDER GOWNS. If you have sexy shoulders, go ahead and flaunt them.

• MAKE YOUR WHOLE SILHOUETTE LOOK LONGER AND LEANER. Try a one-piece structured shape like a sheath or an A-line dress with a fitted bodice and fuller skirt.

• GO OUT OF YOUR COMFORT ZONE WITH COLOR. Experience the slimming benefits of navy, espresso, or pewter used monochromatically.

• TRY TO COMBINE THREE OR MORE FLAW FIGHTERS IN ONE DRESS. For example, a wide V empire dress that's knee length in a solid deep-chocolate color would give you more reasons to buy it.

• GO FOR STRUCTURED COATS AND TUNICS IN RICH FABRICS. You can pull these off. Wear them over narrow silk or crepe pants for evening; over jeans for more casual dress-ups.

BRILLIANT BUYS

FAVORITE FIGURE-FRIENDLY DESIGNERS AND BRANDS FOR EVENING WEAR . . . WHY AND WHERE TO FIND:

ABS by Allen Schwartz (nordstrom.com). For his long, strapless, tiered, and one-shoulder looks, from $228 to $395.

Amsale (bloomingdales.com). For long strapless gowns with ruching in sophisticated colors, from $280 to $990.

Badgley Mischka Platinum Label (saksfifthavenue.com, neimanmarcus.com). For elegant silk chiffons, long and short, from $695 to $1,195.

BCBG Max Azria (saksfifth-avenue.com). For his trend-conscious halters and cut-away shoulders, from $248 to $398.

Calvin Klein Plus Size (macys.com). For the classy LBDs (little black dresses), short and long, in sizes 14–24.

Carmen Marc Valvo (saksfifthavenue.com). For his glam lace, beading, and sequins, and sexy structure, from $395 to $895.

Chetta B (dillards.com, nordstrom.com). For tiered dresses and curve-conscious fits that are not too low cut.

David Meister (saksfifthavenue.com, bloomingdales.com). For his excellent selection of LBDs long and short, V-necks, and sleeves in the $268 to $508 range.

Donna Karan (nordstrom.com). $995. Her jersey dresses drape over every flaw effortlessly and miraculously. Often worn by 40+ actresses on magazine covers.

Heidi Weisel New York (Neiman Marcus). For her understatedly glamorous, simply elegant, body-flattering cocktail dresses.

Kay Unger (saksfifthavenue .com, bloomingdales.com). For her sleeves and perfect-pitch necklines and length.

Laundry by Shelli Segal (bloomingdales.com, nordstrom.com). For the reasonable price of a draped-front, long charmeuse dress, around $295.

Nicole Miller (saksfifthavenue .com). For her muted shimmery fabrics and perfect fit for petites.

Robert Rodriguez (nordstrom .com, saksfifthavenue.com). For his gorgeous fabrics and couture finishing at off-the-rack prices.

Tadashi (nordstrom.com, bloomingdales.com, saksfifthavenue.com). For the off-shoulder ruching, pleating, and dress-plus-bolero thinking.

White House Black Market (whitehouseblackmarket.com). For their great shrugs and LBDs.

FOR A STRAPLESS DRESS

Spanx Hide & Sleek Strapless Full Slip, style 077A, nude or black, $72; Bloomingdale's, spanx.com.

Vows *for* Evening

☐   **I WILL** stop insisting I can merely "change the accessories" and wear the same-old, same-old black pants and top and still look and feel great.

☐   **I WILL** use ruching and draping—not volume—to hide flaws.

☐   **I WILL NOT** buy a size smaller just because it's on sale.

☐   **I WILL** buy the shapewear when I buy the dress.

☐   **I WILL NOT** borrow a dress from my teenage daughter or sister.

☐   **I WILL NOT** shop for party clothes in "emergency" mode.

☐   **I WILL** stock up on foot pads so that I can bare legs in high heels.

☐   **I WILL** carry a small evening clutch when going out at night and leave that heavy workaday tote behind.

DON'T YOU DARE...
Pull out a LBD from ten years ago with the same old accessories and think that you're going to look glam. To stay current, keep up on the trends. In evening right now, look for at least one of the following: Grecian style, draping with jewels, one-shouldered, and dark berry colors or metallics.

16

How to *Never* Look Fat Again

CONGRATULATIONS!

Now you know it all! I hope that from now on, you can intuitively assess your clothes and accessories in terms of high fat and no fat for your body type.

→ You should be very clear about what should remain in your closet and what has to be evicted. And if you're not 100 percent sure, you can always go back and reread the high-fat/no-fat lists. (That's why you need to keep this book on your bedside table!) If you haven't been actively pruning your wardrobe chapter by chapter, the time has come to take action. This is the fun part . . . let's head to your closet and trim the fat! Don't worry, you're not going to have to part with everything you currently own. (All your clothes can't be high fat!) Neither are you going to buy an entirely new wardrobe.

What you want to do is to shop your own closet with your newly trained eye and fresh desire to lighten up, so you see how liberating it can be to actually, physically, remove the heavy emotional baggage lurking in your closet, in your drawers, and on your shelves. You're on your way to getting rid of all your fat clothes.

These clothes are bad for you, so don't think for a second that you should maybe just relocate them to another closet or the basement just in case! You don't want to be tempted to put these on ever again. Why would you ever want to go back to that fat place? You've graduated! You don't need a friend to help you. You don't need a personal shopper. You can be your own personal shopper. Yes, you can!

Some of your pieces can be salvaged with a little assist from your tailor, if they're worth it. Others, which are high fat and unsalvageable, you have to be brave enough to say goodbye to. Send them off into the universe to find another woman with a body type that will actually benefit from wearing them. If you don't shed at least some of your fat clothes, I have to tell you that you wasted your time and money on this book! So come on. Make your investment worth it!

WHAT TO DO WITH
YOUR CAST-OFFS

*If you have good stuff, and the time to deal with an eBay auction,
you could land yourself a nice chunk of change.*

SELL ON EBAY

Auctioning off your pre-worn or never-worn goods on eBay has become a rite of passage for many a fashionista. If you have good stuff, and the time to deal with an eBay auction, you could land yourself a nice chunk of change. If you can't be bothered going through all these steps—taking photos, writing a description, posting the item, organizing the auction, sending it out via post office or UPS (whew!)—there are people who will gladly do the eBay selling for you, and take a well-earned percentage. These saints are called "trading assistants," and you can find them within miles from you on eBay.com. For me, the service they provide is so worth it.

But if you want to do it yourself, eBay style director Constance White has some tips for sellers new to eBay:

LABELS MATTER. Designer labels are your best bet for earning the most cash. Some of the most in-demand names and keywords right now are Ed Hardy, sunglasses, Hollister, and Abercrombie & Fitch. Top brand names also include Michael Kors, Chloe, Manolo Blahnik, Dolce & Gabbana, Cole Haan, Ralph Lauren, Betsey Johnson, and The North Face.

THINK VINTAGE. Vintage items are always hot sellers. But don't limit yourself: Vintage applies to more than just clothes. Think handbags, shoes, pocket watches, charms, rings, and bracelets.

STAY IN SEASON. Sell spring and summer clothes in the summer—when there is the highest demand for them.

AIM HIGH. If you have a precious piece you don't want to part with for less than a certain dollar amount, set a reserve price. Selling should be sweet, not painful!

DO YOUR RESEARCH. Take the time to look online at how similar items have sold. This will give you a good idea of how to price.

TAKE PHOTOGRAPHS. Use a simple white or light-blue background to photograph the item, and shoot it in direct sunlight, or with plenty of indoor lighting. Photograph the front, back, and any details on the item. Spend a half hour Googling "tips for selling on eBay." You will be surprised at the wealth of info available to you.

CREATE STANDOUT TITLES. Use keywords that someone might use when searching for your item: color, size, brand/designer, new.

USE DESCRIPTIVE LISTINGS. Include as much detail as possible: size, measurements if appropriate, color, designer, embellishments, and any and all flaws on the garment.

COMMUNICATE. Potential buyers may ask you additional questions about the item you are selling. Try to answer them promptly and with as much detail as possible.

HOST A CLOTHING SWAP

Without a doubt, the most social way to unload your unwanted clothing and accessories is by hosting or attending a clothing swap. "Clothing swaps are all about quality, not quantity," says Randi Brookman Harris, a freelance prop stylist who hosts these sartorial shindigs seasonally in Manhattan. Her advice is to e-mail your girlfriends and ask them to bring a shopping bag full of pieces that don't work for them anymore. Invite friends who are similar in size or ask them to bring accessories such as handbags, scarves, costume jewelry. "Ideally you want them to bring newish things," she says. "Make sure they know to leave the pit-stained, hole-covered garments at home." Randi puts out a platter of food and organizes everyone's offerings into categories—jackets, skirts, shirts, etc. She lets her friends pick through the goods and try things on at their leisure. No money is exchanged. You can take anything you want and as much as you want. Whatever is left over, the hostess donates to her favorite charity. Maybe you want to be the one to organize your friends (or book club!).

DONATE

Giving your clothing away to someone who will really appreciate it is gratifying. What's high fat on you could be no fat and charming on someone else. You can donate to the Salvation Army, Dress for Success, or Bottomless Closet.

Here's what you need to know if you're going to make a charitable donation to the Salvation Army or a similar organization for a tax deduction.

TAKE PICTURES or write down a detailed description of each item you're donating.

CHECK OUT the Salvation Army Web site's Valuation Guide for realistic dollar amounts for clothing donations (salvationarmyusa.org). These are the amounts you can use—lowest and highest—for write-offs. (Under "Ways to Give," see "Donation Receipts—Valuation Guide.")

GET A STAMPED OR SIGNED RECEIPT when you drop off your goods.

BE SURE TO SAVE THE RECEIPT for your next income tax filing in a place where you can find it when you need it.

> Giving your clothing away to someone who will really appreciate it is gratifying. What's high fat on you could be no fat and charming on someone else.

WORK WITH A CONSIGNMENT SHOP

Before eBay, everyone took unwanted clothes to the consignment shop. If you have a good one close by, call before you make the trip. Some are very picky in what they'll take. Places like Tokyo Joe and Ina in New York City only accept luxe designer brands, and they have to be in keeping with the season. Know ahead of time that many of them take up to 50 percent of the resale, and you have to check in with them to see if your items have sold. If you can't be bothered, just donate to charity. ●

If I Knew These 37 Things Sooner, I Would Be Thinner

Some women will do anything to be thin. I'm not one of them. I'd rather follow the rules in this book for dressing thin and be a few pounds over my ideal weight than do anything unhealthy. When I heard what models were allegedly eating backstage at the New York fashion shows—cotton balls soaked in orange juice in order to stay full!—I decided that I should probably share what works for me. I'm no doctor, but I have to assume that any of the following is preferable than downing a dozen cotton balls!

(1)

See a doctor or a nutritionist to find out the number of calories you need to eat a day to lose weight—and to maintain your weight. If you don't know this, you don't really know how much you can eat. You can also look online or get one of the many books on nutrition to figure out your specifics.

(2)

Weigh yourself first thing in the morning, before coffee. When you weigh yourself, take off everything, even your watch and earrings. Some nutritionists and doctors say not to weigh yourself daily, but how else do you know how you did yesterday? And what you need to do today?

(3)

Eat whole grains for breakfast. Oatmeal with cinnamon and skim milk is very filling.

(4)

Buy a little food diary or use the free iPhone app, "Lose It." Record everything you eat. "If you nibble, you have to scribble," is what I learned in Weight Watchers.

(5)

Calculate your calories as they occur. Don't wait till the end of the day or you may have gone over your limit.

(6)

Measure everything you eat in measuring cups or with a scale—blueberries, salmon, etc.

(7)

Don't let fattening foods enter your home, and you won't be tempted. Walking around with a cart in a grocery store is when you have to be most disciplined.

(8)

Buy small packs if you can't control yourself. For example, buy ice cream sandwiches instead of a box of ice cream or snack boxes of raisins instead of a large container.

(9)

It's said that people who consume 100 to 1,400 milligrams of calcium a day actually lose more weight. You need to consume calcium to keep bones strong anyway, so this is another motivator. It's hard to get enough without supplements, so try the chocolate ones! Just count the calories.

(10)

If you receive a fattening gift—cookies, chocolates, brownies—pack it up and bring it to the office, or give it to the next person you run into.

(11)

If you don't know what to have for dinner, make a dish of roasted veggies: Brussels sprouts, eggplant, asparagus, onions, red pepper with a couple of teaspoons of olive oil at 400 degrees for a half hour.

(12)

Move your body every day. If you can't do a proper workout, then at least walk to a place you would normally drive. Or walk up and down steps instead of taking an elevator at work or home.

(13)

If you haven't a clue what to eat for lunch, boil an egg or two.

(14)

Next time you reach for a diet cola, ask yourself, "Would I be just as satisfied with a glass of water?"

(15)

Don't eat when you're sitting in front of the TV or computer. You'll lose track of what's going into your mouth.

(16)

Try not to eat when you're in transit—leaving the house, in the car, walking on the street—it just looks bad, and you can wait.

(17)

Don't bake unless you intend to give your baked goodies away or bring them somewhere within the hour.

(18)

Put cinnamon on everything you can. It burns calories and adds spice.

(19)

Don't wear elastic pants—you'll never know what your real weight is.

(20)

Listen to music when you're working out. People who do work out longer.

(21)

If you're wearing comfy shoes, you will be more likely to walk. Carry a pair in your bag or in your car.

(22)

Anything less than ten blocks, consider walking.

(23)

Buy an oil spritzer so you spray on just a little olive oil, instead of pouring on a lot.

(24)

Floss or brush your teeth after each meal. When your teeth are clean, you're less likely to eat more food.

(25)

An avocado a day is not a good idea. Once in a while, they are a great treat, but too many are the pits when counting calories.

(26)

Save yourself a little cushion of calories—130 or so—so you can "cheat" on something at the end of the day.

(27)

When you open the door of the fridge for the fifteenth time that day, ask yourself, "Am I really hungry?" If the answer is no, pour yourself a glass of water, shut the door, and leave the kitchen.

(28)
One banana a day is plenty.

(29)
A box of dates contains enough calories for the entire day.

(30)
Even if the bag of popcorn is by a healthy food company, a huge bag could be more calories than your average dinner.

(31)
Licking the spoon or bowl when you're making cookies or cakes counts in your daily calories.

(32)
Reduced-fat peanut butter is still fattening!

(33)
All granola bars are not created equal; in fact, some are super-fattening. My nutritionist, Jennifer Andrus, recommended the brand GNU, which I love in cinnamon raisin.

(34)
Chew your food. Try fifty times before you swallow. The slower you eat, the less you eat.

(35)
"After eight, gain weight." Try not to eat after 8 p.m. Close the kitchen for the night after dinner, and don't go back in.

(36)
Keep your mind engaged. Many times we walk into the kitchen and open the refrigerator out of sheer boredom.

(37)
Try not to make every social activity revolve around food. See a movie instead of having dinner. Take an exercise class or walk or get a massage instead of lunching.

The **100** *Most Fattening Things You Can Wear*

You don't have to spend a bundle to look Fit Not Fat.
It doesn't cost you anything to toss these!

1. Acid-washed jeans

2. Ankle-strap shoes

3. Après-ski boots

4. Baby-doll dress

5. Backpacks

6. Ballerina skirts

7. Ballet flats

8. Balloon hemlines

9. Bear-like, full-length fur coat

10. Belly bracelets

11. Bikinis

12. Birkenstocks

13. Boatneck sailor-stripe tops

14. Boxy blazers

15. Bright turtlenecks

16. Caftans

17. Caged shoes

18. Capped sleeves

19. Capri pants

20. Cargo pants

21. Cartoon sweaters, tees, and PJs

22. Chalet ski sweaters

23. Chokers that choke you

24. Circle skirts

25. Classic pastel twinsets

26. Clip-on button earrings

27. Crazy-colored tights

28. Crew-neck sweaters

29. Crocs!

30. Across-the-body messenger and shoulder bags

31. Cuffed pants

32. Cut-offs and Daisy Dukes

33. Down vests

34. Drawstring waist pants

35. Drindl skirts

36. Elastic-waist pants, including sweatpants

37. Elizabethan ruffle blouses

38. Fanny packs

39. Fisherman sweaters

40. Five-inch-wide belts

41. Flip-flops

42. Floral pants

43. Fur or faux chubbies (stoles)

44. Gladiator sandals

45. Handbags as big as luggage

46. High-waist pants

47. High-waist skirts

48. Holiday-themed sweaters

49. Horizontal zebra stripes

50. Hot pants

51. Jodhpurs

52. Jumpsuits

53. Knit jackets

54. Lace-up espadrilles

55. Leather pants

56. Leg warmers

57. Maxi puffer coats

58. Micro-mini dresses and skirts

59. Mom jeans

60. Newsboy caps

61. Origami-folded dresses

62. Orthopedic-looking shoes

63. Overalls

64. Over-the-knee boots

65. Oversized sweatshirts

66. Oversized T-shirts

67. Patch-pocket shirts

68. Peasant skirts

69. Penny loafers

70. Plaid anything

71. Pleated pants

72. Pleated skirts

73. Pucci print dresses

74. Ripped jeans

75. Round eyewear

76. Safari jackets

77. Scrunchies and banana clips

78. Second-skin pants or jeans

79. Sequin muscle T-shirts

80. Shirtdresses

81. Shorts—boy, girl, Bermuda

82. Shoulder pads

83. Shrunken baby T-shirts

84. Sneakers with jeans

85. Stockings with big patterns

86. Stockings with seams

87. Stretched-out bras

88. Super-wide fishnets

89. Tent dresses

90. Thick platform shoes

91. Thick, wide headbands

92. Tie-dyed anything

93. Tube tops and bustiers

94. UGGs

95. Waist-high granny panties

96. Waist-high nude hose

97. White coats

98. White pants

99. White shoes

100. White stockings

Raise your hand if you think you look fat. You're not alone. Almost every woman I know thinks she does—even those who exercise every day, eat nothing but salads and salmon, and wear a size six or less!

—Charla Krupp, from the Introduction

All women want to look thinner and chicer, but are constantly sabotaged by their clothes. Style expert Charla Krupp, best-selling author of *How Not to Look Old,* knows: It's not you, it's your clothes! If you stop wearing things that make you look heavier than you actually are, you can look thinner by *tonight*—without starving, exercising, or doing anything crazy.

In HOW TO *NEVER* LOOK FAT AGAIN, Charla has devised a fresh, fast, and simple way to determine whether a piece of clothing is going to pack on the pounds. All you have to do is think about each item you wear in terms of how fattening it is. Simply steer clear of high fat clothes—those guaranteed to make you look flabby and frumpy—and wear no-fat as often as you can. How simple is that?

You'll never get dressed the same way again once you discover:

- smart, easy ways to hide arm flap, a big bust, a muffin top, back fat, a Buddha belly, a big booty, wide hips, thunder thighs, heavy calves—and that's only half the book!
- which fabrics, colors, and styles make you look fat—and which ones make the pounds drop away
- clever solutions for special situations—workout gear, evening wear, and even swimsuits!
- Charla's "Brilliant Buys": the brands, fashions, and services that really deliver—and a list of which products to avoid
- the top ten tips for every body issue that will make you look thinner by tonight!

Finally, you can stop asking your husband, girlfriend, boyfriend, sister, brother, mother, coworker: "Does this make me look fat?" Now the answer will always be "No!"

CHARLA KRUPP is a nationally known style expert who appeared for ten years on the *Today* show and on more than thirty national TV shows, including *The Oprah Winfrey Show, The View, The Tyra Banks Show, The Early Show, Entertainment Tonight,* and *Access Hollywood.* Krupp is a contributing editor to *People: Style Watch* and was formerly beauty director at *Glamour,* a senior editor at *InStyle,* and a fashion columnist at *More.* She has written for the *New York Times, TIME,* and many fashion magazines and websites. She lives in New York City and Sagaponack, New York, with her husband, Richard Zoglin.

Skinny Clicks

YOUR GUIDE TO NO FAT SHOPPING ONLINE

For women who are embarrassed to get dressed and undressed in public, the Internet has become a shopping godsend. Shop online, and keep your indignity intact. You avoid the prospect of a dressing room with no mirror, which forces you to step out and catch a glimpse in the communal one. There are also the dreaded communal dressing rooms, and dressing rooms with such skimpy curtains that they might as well be communal. Then again, you may not even have the time to drive to a mall and go shopping. Many women I know prefer to ship merchandise back then to wait in a long checkout line or deal with the attitudes of sales associates. Almost all online retailers have a generous return policy (just check before you enter your credit card number). Ready, set, shop! With this list as your guide, you'll have your new skinny basics in just a few clicks.

24 Hour Fitness

(24hourfitness.com) This is where to buy the BodyBugg Calorie Management System featured on TV's *The Biggest Loser*. This little portable device will basically do everything but slap your wrist when you reach for the cookie jar. It uses a multisensor approach to monitor how many calories you take in versus how many you're burning.

Bare Necessities

(barenecessities.com) Stock your lingerie drawer—from bras to bottoms—at this site. It has all the top brands in underthings, such as Wacoal, TC, Wolford, La Perla, and Hanky Panky. Also find a huge selection of larger sizes from Fantasie.

Be Beautiful

(bebeautiful.com) Find some of my favorite get-gorgeous brands here like Spanx, Essie, and Tweezerman. Their "Outlet" section offers an ever-changing selection of deeply discounted must-haves.

Bloomingdale's

(bloomingdales.com) Who doesn't love Bloomies? The iconic department store's e-commerce site has all the best denim brands, including Not Your Daughter's Jeans, 7 For All Mankind, Citizens of Humanity, and J Brand. Bonus: You can return anything purchased online at one of its retail locations.

Bluefly

(bluefly.com) Bluefly is the biggest virtual sample sale on earth, packed with the world's hottest designers (Christian Louboutin, Prada, Michael Kors, and Shoshanna). You may never pay retail again once the Bluefly bug bites you.

Drugstore.com

(drugstore.com) With brands like Philosophy and Fekkai, it's not your average drugstore. Get, your skin glowing with Jergen's Natural Glow Daily Moisturizer, a staple of every beautyista's cosmetic wardrobe.

Fashion Fit Formula

(fashionfitformula.com) Founders Janet Wood and Kathy McFadden have figured out a way—through a series of mathematical calculations—to make your clothes look the best they possibly can on you. Purchase one of their packages through their site.

Fresh Pair

(freshpair.com) Choose from sexy lingerie to smart shapewear pieces from a plethora of brands, including Le Mystére.

Her Room

(herroom.com) Shop the extensive selection of bras, panties, and stockings from brands such as Olga, Chantelle, La Perla, and Natori.

HSN

(hsn.com) Find all the beauty and fashion brands featured on HSN. Love its selection of RJ Graziano jewelry and Clever Carriage handbags.

J. Crew

(jcrew.com) Classy, chic, and good enough for Michelle Obama. Its selection of swimwear has shapes and colors for every taste.

Lipo in a Box

(lipoinabox.com) Skip the surgery and log onto this site for great shapewear. Founder Connie Elder tackles every problem area with Lipo in a Box's comfy panties, bodysuits, camisoles, and capris. Love that she extended the usual shapewear shades to include chocolate.

Maidenform

(maidenform.com) A wide range of bras at a nice price. Includes full sizes, minimizers, soft cups, back-smoothers, push-ups and strapless. They also have Control It swimwear, which is body-slimming bathing suits that hold in all the mushy bits.

Nordic Track

(nordictrack.com) Nothing beats working out in the privacy of your own home. Aside from treadmills, ellipticals, and exercise bikes, you can shop for workout gear, including sports bras and high-tech jackets.

Nordstrom

(nordstrom.com) Nordstrom has all the big names in fashion plus a terrific selection of Miraclesuit Swimwear ultra-slimming bathing suits.

QVC

(qvc.com) Their all-star product lineup includes beauty goods from makeup artist Mally Roncal and dermatologist Dr. Patricia Wexler. Look for designer Lori Goldstein's LOGO, a collection of embellished T-shirts, leggings, and blazers, cut very generously. Also find Breezies Intimates, a super-soft, moisture-wicking lingerie collection offering full-support bras and panties.

Saks Fifth Avenue

(saksfifthavenue.com) Just as you would expect, this Web site is packed with the best in beauty and fashion.

Sephora

(sephora.com) If you can't pop into one of the beauty giant's entertaining stores, then log onto its site for a generous selection of the best in makeup, skincare, and hair—all very easy to navigate by brand.

Space NK

(spacenk.com) High-quality and often hard-to-find beauty brands populate the virtual shelves of this UK-based beauty retailer that has debuted in select Bloomingdale's stores stateside.

Spanx

(spanx.com) Spanx has changed the face—and the butts, hips, thighs, and calves—of the shapewear industry. If you want to discreetly hide bulges, lumps and bumps, go to this site for its entire line, including Haute Contour, and its new slimming swimwear.

Target

(target.com) "Tar-jay" was the first retailer to really understand the concept of fast fashion by hot designers. Target is a must-stop for wallet-conscious fashionistas.

Tres Sleek

(tressleek.com) Compressing your mushy parts is the name of the game at Tres Sleek. Love its special sleeves to banish bat wings.

Victoria's Secret

(victoriassecret.com) Victoria's Secret has become the retailer to beat for a selection of affordable, ever-rotating lingerie trends. Many of the models in this book came to the casting in VS bras!

Zappos

(zappos.com) At last check, Zappos carried over three hundred d'Orsay styles (the most Fit Not Fat shoe out there). From Giuseppe Zanotti and Stuart Weitzman to Marc by Marc Jacobs and Isaac Mizrahi, you'll pretty much find any style, size (including wide widths), and color you're craving. Easy returns.

Skinny Clicks
for Larger Sizes

Big girls, don't cry! The selection keeps getting better,
according to my friend Michele Weston, a fashion authority
who really knows the size 14-and-over market. Some of the
Web sites here are her favorites for curvy women who never
want to forsake style.

Anna Scholz

(annascholz.com) This German designer calls her spring line "curvaceous couture." Her flirty collection of on-trend dresses, trench coats, and tunics are cut in sizes 12–28. Think Michael Kors meets Tahari.

Avenue

(avenue.com) You can't beat the denim selection at this affordable and trendy retailer. Find tunics, swimwear, and dresses in sizes 14–32.

Chadwick's

(chadwicks.com) Chadwick's wins the chic award for stocking its Web site with a wardrobe fit for Audrey Hepburn: jacquard jackets, sheath dresses, and clean-front pants.

Chico's

(chicos.com) Comfortable style is the name of the game at Chico's. Find wrinkle-free separates and a selection of tunics, jackets, and trendy jewelry.

Evans

(evans.co.uk) Cute swimwear, laid-back tees, camisoles, and tanks, and bold printed dresses and tunics from this British retailer.

JCPenney

(jcp.com) You'll find chic pieces in their Bisou Bisou dresses and Worthington brand lines that go up to 24W and 3X. And they're not afraid to show bigger women on their website. Love that.

La Grande Dame

(lagrandedame.com) Find an uber-chic selection of dresses from David Meister and Olivia Harper, jeans from James Jeans and Not Your Daughter's Jeans, and separates from De Sentino and Zen Knits. You can also shop by body type, occasion, or trend.

Lane Bryant

(lanebryant.com) When you want great-looking basics, hit this plus-sized leader. They also offer an extensive array of fun and sexy lingerie from Cacique and shapewear from Spanx.

Macy's

(macys.com) Find a multitude of plus-sized choices from Tommy Hilfiger, Michael by Michael Kors, and INC, plus its in-house line, Style & Co.

Neiman Marcus

(neimanmarcus.com) A great resource for sizes 14 and up, Neiman's online has hip jeans, dresses, shirts, and skirts from plus-size designers, including Anna Scholz, Melissa Masse, XCVI, Eileen Fisher, and more.

One Stop Plus

(onestopplus.com) Billing itself as "the online fashion mall for plus sizes," it literally is one-stop shopping for the curvy customer. Find everything from formal wear to sleepwear. Brand boutiques within the site include such designers as Taillissime, Jessica London, Ellos, and Roaman's.

Ralph Lauren

(ralphlauren.com) Shop for Lauren by Ralph Lauren. RL's preppy chic collection goes up to size 18.

Walmart

(walmart.com) A Norma Kamali wrap dress for $20? Wide-leg jersey pants for $18? Kudos to Kamali for her chic collection up to size XXL.

Zaftique

(zaftique.com) You'll be hard pressed to find a better selection of dresses for formal and semi-formal occasions anywhere else. Zaftique's jewel-toned frocks come in every style under the sun.

THANK YOUS

FIRST OFF, thank you to my brilliant and supportive editor, the phenomenal Karen Murgolo, editorial director of the Springboard Press at Grand Central Publishing, who went to great lengths to make this a breakthrough book. I was not interested in doing a style guide that resembled any other, and fortunately, neither was Karen. Our partnership is heaven because we are totally in sync about what we, as women, want to read.

A ZILLION THANKS to Jamie Raab, publisher of Grand Central Publishing. Behind every successful book is a genius publisher who makes all the right decisions every step of the way. I'm forever grateful that Jamie, was there for me since the conception of this book, with her unwavering, 110 percent, enthusiastic support.

SO HAPPY TO HAVE MY AGENT, the cool-headed Richard Pine, in my corner. He not only got me, but he got the big picture, without prompting. Elisa Petrini, also of InkWell Management, has my deepest appreciation for helping me to navigate the challenging aspects of production. Thanks also to Nathaniel Jacks of InkWell.

THE BEAUTY OF THIS BOOK speaks to the elegance, taste, and creative vision of Eric Hoffman. The visual bar was raised the minute Eric signed on to design the book. I so appreciate Eric for not only his talent but also for being so accommodating, gracious, and caring throughout. The entire team at Hoffman Creative contributed to the look of the book: Stacy Barnes, Benjamin Miller, Tracy Engelhardtsen, and Vanessa Ly. And thanks to Stephenie Fernandez and Ann Taylor at Stardust Vision for their early support.

IN THE WORLDS OF FASHION/BEAUTY, Lois Johnson can do it all and she did for this book. From bouncing off ideas to writing, styling, casting, producing, Lois was always there for me, the very definition of a great girlfriend.

FOR FINDING THE WORDS—AND FAST, many thanks to writer Melissa Schweiger. Melissa and Lois helped me bring these chapters to life, doing the initial heavy lifting with their fashion/beauty expertise and stylish prose.

POP! FLASH! Once again, a big kiss to photographer and cover genius Michael Waring, for the time and dedication he put in to make the cover photo something I am proud of. I can't thank you enough, Michael, for making me look Fit Not Fat! On this cover dream team: the exceptional makeup artist Nick Barose, who made time on his celeb-packed schedule; Arturo of Arturo New York, who always gives cover-worthy hair even at the crack of dawn; and Lois Johnson, for her styling savvy and moral support.

THE DISCERNING EYE of photographer Timothy Hogan made all the model shots worth the price of the book. No matter how many words are used to describe an outfit, nothing compares with seeing it captured to perfection in a stunning photograph. I so appreciate the enormous effort and attentive focus that Tim and his team—Dario Diovisalvi, Bridget Fleming, Andrew Segreti, and Alex Kaed—brought to this book.

I HIT THE JACKPOT with stylist Eve Feuer. Smart and unflappable, she instinctively knows what's high fat and no fat and where to get it by tomorrow. I loved how she styled the models, in accessible yet aspirational looks that real women can relate to. Big thanks to Sarah Benge for all the long hours assisting.

THE FEARLESS MODELS on these pages agreed to flaunt their least flattering body parts in pursuit of a higher goal and, in doing so, inspire us all to seek that level of confidence, comfort, and pride about our bodies. You rock! Loved working with Casey McCabe, Lizzie Miller, Bernadett Vajda, Michelle Griffin from Wilhemina as well as Elizabeth Green and Maiysha Simpson from Ford.

TWO AMAZING FRIENDS of mine read and critiqued every chapter. My sharp as a whip friend Abby Ross of Miami, who has been a serious Weight Watcher for most of her life, poured over the early manuscript. Additional gratitude to Abby for dragging me into the digital age; in the world of social media, Abby is queen.

KUDOS TO SUSAN TOEPFER. I had the good fortune of having the editorial expertise of one of the best editors in the magazine business do an edit of the final manuscript. With her sharp editorial eye, Susan made improvements to every page.

CREATING BUZZ for a book takes a village. I am fortunate to have the best in the biz in-house at Grand Central Publishing. Thanks to the savvy Matthew Ballast, for masterfully calling the shots. I so appreciate the unstoppable support of Tanisha Christie, who goes above and beyond. The terrific Melissa Bullock is always there for me on the other end of the e-mail.

AND AT FLYING TELEVISION, big thanks to Lori Levine and Alexa Susser.

ALSO AT GRAND CENTRAL PUBLISHING, the team that lent their expert two cents to the production of this book included Diane Luger, who tremendously influenced the cover; Tareth Mitch, for her expert production editing; Philippa White for her can-do good attitude and all-around helpfulness; Pam Schechter and Vidya Thanabal, who worked wonders with the printing; and to Suzanne Albert, Nicole Bond, and Peggy Boelke, who all helped get the book into the right hands.

BLOOMINGDALE'S, THE ULTIMATE FASHION CLOSET, provided one-stop shopping for most of the no-fat clothes. For this, I can't say thanks enough to my fabulous friend, Anne Keating, the senior vice president of Bloomingdale's public relations, who always makes things happen; as well as Frank Doroff, Bloomingdale's vice chairman of ready to wear. It's a pleasure working with Anne's A-team of PR pros: Lori Griffith, Liz McGovern, Ashley Bechard, Sasha Soyfer, Nancy Lueck, Mara Maddox,

Peggy Lanigan, Sara Nix, Wanda Ahmadi, Jaime Strong, Dana Weiss, Nancy Peck, Alexandra Karcev, Jamie A Habanek, and Emilie Marvosa.

ADDITIONAL WARDROBE provided by the following. A special thanks to my friends in fashion who generously sent clothes, shapewear, stockings, shoes, and accessories for photography.

Joni Fischer of Christopher Fischer

Maggie Adams of Spanx

Lori Ann Robinson of Lori Ann Robinson Consultants

David Welsch of TC shapewear

Lisa Stein of LA Stein

Sharyn Soleimani of Barneys New York,

Wendy Converse and RJ Graziano of RJ Graziano

Leslie Stevens of LaForce & Stevens for Wacoal

Denise Skelton and Dan Sackrowitz of barenecessities.com.

Connie Elder of Lipo-in-a-Box

Michelle Smith and Lauren Atterman of Milly

Anna Natsume and Robert Marc of Robert Marc

Dana Chinitz of Stuart Weitzman

Della Olsher and Erica Levine of D&E marketing

Rachel Kapor at KH Public Relations for Asics

Whitney DeLear at Calvin Klein

Kristen Raymaakers at Mullen for Saucony

Ann Magnin at Magnin PR for Panache

King Chong at Lafayette148

Megan Oxland at Magaschoni

Saulo Villela at Adrienne Landau

Alison Hessert at Hue

Nicole Lando at Alison Brod Public Relations for Hanky Panky

FRIENDS IN THE BEAUTY BIZ, you know who you are. Thanks for the latest in lipsticks, eyeshadows, primers, and plumpers, etc. Couldn't have found those Brilliant Buys without all of you.

LOUD SHOUT OUT to Lisa Gabor. We had the good fortune of having our offices at *InStyle* next to each other, and since we were often the only ones there on Saturdays, we bonded over big ideas and have been collaborating ever since. Her genius is matched only by her ginormous generosity of spirit.

FRIENDS AND FAMILY who always come through for me, whether road-testing beauty products, hosting a book signing, spending the weekend trying on shapewear, showing up at a book event, etc. Kim Isaacsohn; Laurette Kittle; Cindy Lewis; Della Olsher; Cynthia Parsons; Jane Berk; Lisa Glinsky; Barbara Graustark; Amy Schwartz; Lora Nasby; Katie Couric; Charlie Esposito; Julie Weinstein Sacchetta, Terry, Jay, Lisa, Mollie, Jami Krupp; Rose, Janet, Larry, Paul Zoglin.

EVERY AUTHOR SHOULD HAVE THE LUXURY of an expert editor—in-house! Thanks to my husband, Richard, for always helping me take it up a notch. While living with a super thin guy makes it pretty near impossible to stay on a diet, buying the High Fat and No Fat version of everything from ice cream to peanut butter to jelly to milk, proved inspirational.

THE PROFESSIONAL EXPERTISE of friends who gave me great advice along the way is so appreciated. These people really know pretty much everyone and everything: Gloria Appel, Larry

Appel, Janet Gurwitch, Camille MacDonald, Mary Mayotte, Debi Fine, Sandi Mendelsohn, Adam Glassman.

BUCKETS OF GRATITUDE to Jaime Wolf, not only my lawyer but also my business guru and copywriter, too! Your intelligence, advice, and due diligence are things I can't live without.

MY FABULOUS ASSISTANTS who helped me with everything from researching to blogging to (dare I say it) Facebook. These impressive journalists include: Sara Gaynes, Karina Martinez-Carter, Carlye Wisel, Alysa Teichman; and most of all, Sara Anderson, who logged in many long hours expertly fact-checking the manuscript. Special thanks to the super-organized Brette Polin, who has always been there for me since our days at *Shop, Etc.*

ONCE AGAIN, I would like to acknowledge my unending gratitude to Judy Linden of the Stonesong Press without whom I wouldn't have made the smooth transition from magazines to books. She changed my life!

MAKEUP! HAIR! CLOTHES! Makeup artist Julie Tussey not only performs magic on me, but could teach a master class on cosmetic technology with all her insider info. We spent a day together smearing, dabbing, blotting, and editing down the best of the Brilliant Buys.

HAIR COLOR GENIUS Brad Johns of New York's Red Door Salon and Spa, who has been blonding me forever, has a point of view on everything, including how not to look fat with your hair color!

CHRIS CUSANO, also of New York's Red Door Salon and Spa, is the master of precision, who has been cutting my hair since forever. He gave me the bangs and chic cut on display in these pages.

IT WAS A REAL PLEASURE working with stylist Ann Caruso on my outfits. She lives up to her reputation as a class act with a great eye for fashion.

THANKS TO OUR ON-SET BEAUTY PROS, makeup artist Christina Reyna and hairdressers Carmel Bianco and David Cruz. They knew their High Fat from No Fat.

AT TIME INC, my home in the magazine world, two people very special to me are editor-in-chief Martha Nelson, the smartest editor in the magazine industry, with whom I've worked since the early days of *InStyle.* And the fabulous Susan Kaufman, managing editor of the super successful startup, *People: StyleWatch,* which I'm happy to be a part of.

LET'S HAVE A ROUND OF APPLAUSE to the many experts who contributed their time, their insider's secrets, their gold so that we never look fat again! I owe them big-time! XX

Tracy Anderson
Bill Bartlett
Oscar Blandi
Nancy Boas
Randi Brookman Harris
Tory Burch

Misty Elliott
Dr. Gervaise Gerstner
Dr. Jeff Golub-Evans
Kim Isaacsohn
Brad Johns
Dr. Michael Kane
Dr. Suzanne Levine
Dr. Alan Matarasso
Dr. Seth Matarasso
Vicky McGarry
Stella Mikhail
Susan Nethero
Dr. Pamela Peeke
Renee Raimondi

Mally Roncal
Dr. David Rosenberg
Dr. Deborah Sarnoff
Dr. Eric S. Schweiger
Liz Smith
Susan Sommers
Essie Weingarten
Eugenia Weston
Eden Wexler
Constance White
Abby Z.
Ruth Zukerman

ONE LAST THANK YOU, to all the fashion designers who make chic clothes for women size 14 and up: please know that you have made a tremendous impact on women's lives. To all designers who don't cut beyond size 12, I say, continue to do so at your own peril. In a down economy, turning your backs on more than half of all women in this country doesn't sound like a plan. Neither does it sound fashionable when inclusiveness is in the zeitgeist. Let's not deny all women the chance to dress well whatever their size (or age). Amen.

FASHION CREDITS

Here's where we found all our non-fat clothes. Please realize that items available at press time may no longer be available, because fashion changes seasonally. But knowing the brand and retailer may help when curating your own no-fat wardrobe.

COVER

Christopher Fischer cashmere "Gisele" open front cardigan. Underneath, cotton, three-quarter sleeve V-neck. Both at christopher fischer.com. Habitual Jeans, at Bloomingdale's. Lisa Stein 18k white-gold crystal and diamond pendants on 18k white-gold white-sapphire chain, and 18k diamond-studded hoops, all at Jeffrey New York, or see lastein.com for stores.

INTRO

Tory Burch sweater, Bergdorf Goodman, New York. Pencil skirt by Theory, Bergdorf Goodman, New York. Lisa Stein 18k white-gold crystal and diamond pendant on 18k white-gold white-sapphire chain, Jeffrey New York, or see lastein.com for stores.

CHAPTER 2 WIDE FACE

NO FAT, PAGE 27

Cream V-neck sweater by Sutton Studio, Bloomingdale's, blooming dales.com. Gold earrings, Kara, by Kara Ross, Bloomingdale's.

CHAPTER 3 THICK NECK + BROAD SHOULDERS

OPENER, PAGE 36

Cream shawl collar sweater by Ralph Lauren, Bloomingdale's. Yellow-gold "Petal" hoops with marquis diamonds by Lisa Stein, Jeffrey New York, or lastein.com for stores.

NO FAT, PAGE 45

Gray trouser by Calvin Klein, Bloomingdale's. Black scoop neck tank by Elie Tahari, Bloomingdale's. Gray cardigan sweater by Tory Burch, Bloomingdale's. Silver chains and bracelet by RJ Graziano, 212-685-1248. Silver earrings by ABS, Bloomingdale's.

CHAPTER 4 ARM FLAP

OPENER, PAGE 52

Lace Couture Camisole by Spanx Haute Contour, Bloomingdale's. Gold bangles by RJ Graziano, 212-685-1248. Diamond stud earrings, Bloomingdale's.

NO FAT, PAGE 63

White blouson top by Diane von Furstenberg, Bloomingdale's. Bracelets by RJ Graziano, 212-685-1248. Gold bejeweled earring, Bloomingdale's. Jeans (model's own).

CHAPTER 5 BIG BUST

OPENER, PAGE 70

Pink lace bra by Harlequin, barenecessities.com. Silver diamond necklace by RJ Graziano, 212-685-1248.

NO FAT, PAGE 77

Jacket by Lafayette148, lafay ette148.com. Cream V-neck sweater, Sutton Studio, Bloom-ingdale's, bloomingdales.com. Gray skirt by Calvin Klein, Bloom-ingdale's. Gray python pump by Stuart Weitzman, stuartweitzman .com. Lisa Stein 18k white-gold crystal and diamond pendant on 18k white-gold white-sapphire chain, Jeffrey New York, or see lastein.com for stores.

CHAPTER 6 MUFFIN TOP + BACK FAT

OPENER, PAGE 86

White Lycra® bathing suit, by LaBlanca, by Rod Beattie, Bloomingdale's.

NO FAT, PAGE 95

Dark-wash denim by Ralph Lauren, Bloomingdale's. Purple cotton Elie Tahari shirt, Bloomingdale's. Leather belt by Hobo, Bloomingdale's. Gold bangles by RJ Graziano, 212-685-1248.

CHAPTER 7 BUDDHA BELLY

OPENER, PAGE 100

Magenta lace tank and bikini brief by Hanky Panky, hankypanky.com.

NO FAT, PAGE 109

Black V-neck dress by Hugo Boss, Bloomingdale's. Black peep-toe pumps by Stuart Weitzman, stuart weitzman.com. Leather belt by Hobo, Bloomingdale's. Gold cuff by Aqua, at Bloomingdale's. Gold hoop earrings by ABS, Bloomingdale's. Watch by Longines. Black crocodile clutch by Clever Carriage, clever carriagecompany.com.

CHAPTER 8 WIDE HIPS + THIGHS

OPENER, PAGE 114

Gray cashmere shorts by Christopher Fischer, christopherfischer .com. Coral scoop neck tank by Elie Tahari, available at Bloomingdale's.

NO FAT, PAGE 123

Black pencil skirt by Hugo Boss, Bloomingdale's. White button-front shirt by Theory, Bloomingdales. Black leather pumps (model's own). Black leather bag by Tory Burch, Bloomingdale's. Gold cuffs by RJ Graziano, 212-685-1248.

CHAPTER 9 BIG BOOTY

OPENER, PAGE 128

Nude with ivory lace cami and brief by Wacoal, Bloomingdale's.

NO FAT, PAGE 137

Dark-wash denim, The Essential Jean by Gap. White cotton tank by Elie Tahari, Bloomingdale's. Brown braided-leather heel by Ralph Lauren, Bloomingdale's.

CHAPTER 10 HEAVY CALVES

OPENER, PAGE 142

Black pencil skirt by Hugo Boss, Bloomingdale's. Pink patent leather pumps by Guess, Bloomingdale's. Silver grid-print cuff by Rebecca, Bloomingdale's.

NO FAT, PAGE 151

Leopard print skirt by Lafayette148, lafayette148.com. Black leather pump by Stuart Weitzman, stuartweitzman.com. Spanx Tight-End Tights, spanx.com.

CHAPTER 11 WIDE FEET + ANKLES

OPENER, PAGE 156

Bejeweled zipper heels by Giuseppe Zanotti, zappos.com. On toes, Essie nail color in Wicked, at Ulta.

NO FAT, PAGE 165

Gray pencil skirt by Calvin Klein, Bloomingdale's. Nude pump by Type Z, zappos.com.

CHAPTER 12 SUMMER

OPENER, PAGE 170

Printed chiffon cover-up by Diane von Furstenberg, Bloomingdale's. Brown one-piece bathing suit by Fantasie, barenecessities.com. Gold wedge sandals by Giuseppe Zanotti, Bloomingdale's. Straw hat by Hat Attack, hatattack.com. Cocktail ring by Kara Ross, Bloomingdale's. Bangles by RJ Graziano, 212-685-1248.

NO FAT, PAGE 179

Black Miraclesuit, barenecessities .com. Sandals by Rafe, rafe.com. Sunglasses by Marc Jacobs, marcjacobs.com. Silver hoops by Bloomingdale's, bloomingdales.com. White leather bag by Anya Hindmarch, anyahindmarch.com.

CHAPTER 13 WINTER

OPENER, PAGE 186

Gray sweater with fur collar by Magaschoni, magaschoni.com. Silver fox trapper hat by Adrienne Landau, adriennelandau.com. Gray fur trim scarf by Magaschoni, magaschoni.com. Gray gloves by Magaschoni, magaschoni.com.

NO FAT, PAGE 195

Black evening coat with jeweled buttons by Lafayette148, lafay ette148.com. Black leather boots by Stuart Weitzman, stuartweitzman .com.Tight End Tights by Spanx at spanx.com. Cream cashmere scarf by Christopher Fischer, christopher fischer.com. Knitted Rex rabbit hat by Adrienne Landau, adriennelan-dau.com.

CHAPTER 14 WORKOUT

OPENER, PAGE 200

Graphic tank by Zobha, Bloom-ingdale's. Black yoga pant by Zobha, Bloomingdale's.

NO FAT, PAGE 207

Navy yoga pant by Zobha, Bloom-ingdale's. Navy zip jacket by Zobha, Bloomingdale's. Pink Versatility Cami Sport Tank by New Balance, newbalance.com. Progrid Hurricane sneakers by Saucony, saucony.com.

CHAPTER 15 THE EVENING

OPENER, PAGE 212

Pink one-shoulder cocktail dress by Tadashi, Bloomingdale's. Cocktail ring by Philippe Audibert, Bloom-ingdale's. Crystal evening clutch by Judith Leiber.

NO FAT, PAGE 221

Black chiffon ruffle-front cocktail dress by Tadashi, Bloomingdale's. Pink satin pump by Sergio Rossi, zappos.com. Bracelet by RJ Gra-ziano, 212-685-1248. Earrings by RJ Graziano, 212-685-1248.

CHAPTER 16 HOW TO NEVER LOOK FAT AGAIN

NO FAT, PAGE 228

Purple Derek Lam dress, Barneys New York. Nude patent Manolo Blanik pumps, Bergdorf Goodman, New York. Necklace by RJ Gra-ziano, 212-685-1248.

PHOTOGRAPHY CREDITS

All model photography by Timothy Hogan except for the following: